TALKING SEX...

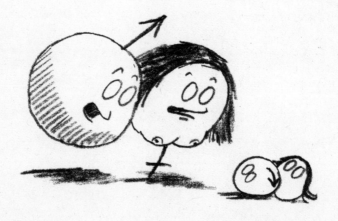

by Lois B. Morris

with your kids

Based on the television program
produced by Tuscany Productions, Inc.,
for Home Box Office

HBO

Illustrated by Tom Sloan

A FIRESIDE BOOK
Published by Simon & Schuster, Inc.
New York

Also by Lois B. Morris

THE LITTLE BLACK PILL BOOK
(coauthor)
THE PILL BOOK OF HEADACHES
(coauthor)

A Fireside Book
Published by Simon & Schuster, Inc.
Simon & Schuster Building
Rockefeller Center
1230 Avenue of the Americas
New York, New York 10020

FIRESIDE and colophon are registered trademarks of
Simon & Schuster, Inc.

Designed by Levavi & Levavi
Manufactured in the United States of America
10   9   8   7   6   5   4   3   2   1

Library of Congress Cataloging in Publication Data

Morris, Lois B.
    Talking sex—with your kids.

    "Based on the television program produced by
Tuscany Production, Inc., for home box office"—
    "A Fireside book."
    Bibliography: p.
    1.Sex instruction.   I.Talking sex—with your
kids (Television program)   II.Title.
HQ57.M67   1984   649'.65   84-14059

ISBN 0-671-50022-8

Acknowledgments

Special thanks to the creative team selected by Tuscany Productions for the "Talking Sex . . . with Your Kids" television program: Kit Laybourne, James R. McGee, Paul and Helena Fierlinger, Stuart Dworeck, and Nan Cinnater. Without their successful efforts, no book would ever have followed.

Thanks to Joan Shigekawa and Angela Solomon for their faith in me and their hard work and serious laughter on the book's behalf.

To Sheila Nevins, the executive whose creative vision, humor, and candor inspired us to produce "Talking Sex . . . with Your Kids," the television program that inspired this book.

Contents

Seventeen Questions—Complete with Answers—to Use When Talking Sex ... with Your Kids:

Preface

Why do parents today need help in discussing sex—a subject that is constantly being exposed in movies, on television and radio, and in magazines?

Experts agree that hearing or reading about a sensitive subject doesn't make it easier to talk about it. Most parents have had very little experience in talking about sex with their parents or teachers. Many couples even find it difficult to talk about sex with each other.

Until recently, sex was a forbidden subject. In many homes it was never mentioned at all. There was no opportunity to share the many feelings that constitute our attitudes about sexuality. So why should we bring up the subject with our children? The answer is that ignorance is *not* bliss. Never talking about sex is a form of sex education too.

A recent study of young parents demonstrates that it is still not easy for them to talk about this subject, despite the information explosion about human sexuality. Fears persist. Fear of conveying the wrong point of view. Fear of the sexual impulse itself. Fear of exposing one's own discomfort. Fear of overemphasizing the importance of sex.

But sex is not only a physical act. Our sexuality is also the way we feel about ourselves as male and female. It is the way we relate to other people and is an integral part of our total personality. Our children are

9

taught about sexuality and love from their very first days—in the way we hold them, touch them, love them.

Parents make the best sex educators, especially if they are knowledgeable, comfortable, and "askable." Children want to hear what their parents have to say, and they will pay close attention to how they say it. I am certain this book will contribute to that learning experience. If it helps you to relax and talk about sex, even with a twinkle in your eye, it will convey something very positive and special to your children about their sexuality.

Talking Sex . . . with Your Kids is an outgrowth of an enormously popular television program, produced by Tuscany Productions for Home Box Office. I was pleased to be able to collaborate on the show in my role, at the time, as president of the American Association of Sex Educators, Counselors, and Therapists (AASECT), the largest professional organization in the field of human sexuality.

Now, I and a team of leading AASECT members are honored to take up this brand-new challenge: to contribute to making *Talking Sex . . . with Your Kids* a book for the whole family to learn from and to enjoy. We hope that as parents you, too, will feel proud of what you can contribute to your child's sexual health.

DR. SHIRLEY ZUSSMAN

Introduction

If there's one common denominator for all parents, it may be the uncertainty they feel when talking about sex and sexual situations with their own kids.

It is not only what to say and how to bring it up in front of the children that is the big stumbling block for parents, but also what you do *not* say that creates an impact.

This book is designed to take the hassle out of talking sex and to help you get your message across as a natural part of everyday living. Sex is perfectly natural and kids are naturally curious—especially about sex—but it is sometimes difficult for parents to remember that when it comes to talking sex with their children.

The American Association of Sex Educators, Counselors, and Therapists (AASECT) has assisted in assembling an extraordinary group of experts to answer your questions about talking sex with your kids. All six experts have made major contributions to the human sexuality field as educators, therapists, authors—and of course as parents.

Carol Cassell, Ph.D., is the current president of AASECT and the former director of education for Planned Parenthood Federation of America. She has traveled to nearly every state giving speeches and presentations and making guest appearances on TV and radio on matters concerning the role of parents in the sex education of their children; teenage sexuality and pregnancy; and sex education in school, church, and community. Her new book, *Swept Away: Why Women Fear Their Own Sexuality*, is about the aftermath of the sexual revolution, and why relationships between men and women are marked by such passion and paradox. Dr. Cassell has four children and lives in Albuquerque, New Mexico.

Lyman Gilmore, Ed.D., father of two, is professor of education at New England College in Henniker, New Hampshire, where he teaches courses in human sexuality, adolescent psychology, and teacher education. He also has a private counseling practice and conducts workshops, seminars, and courses on such subjects as teen sexuality, sexual dysfunction, and sexuality education for parents throughout New Hampshire.

Harold Lief, M.D., is professor of psychiatry at the University of Pennsylvania School of Medicine and psychiatrist to the Pennsylvania Hospital. When he was director of the Center for the Study of Sex Education in Medicine, he fought hard—and successfully—for the introduction of sex education into medical schools. He is a consultant to the Masters-Johnson Institute in St. Louis. Dr. Lief has won numerous awards for his work (including AASECT's Annual Award in 1980), has published widely—and is the father of five children.

Patricia Schreiner-Engel, Ph.D., also has five children. She is assistant professor in the department of psychiatry at the Mount Sinai School of Medicine in New York and is assistant director of the Human Sexuality Program there. For over a decade she has served as director of training and supervising psychologist of

Community Sex Information in New York City. Dr. Schreiner-Engel has a private practice and lectures and conducts workshops on sexuality throughout the United States and Canada.

Mary Lee Tatum, M.Ed., is a nationally recognized leader of sex education in the public schools. She is a teacher in the family life and sex education program of the Falls Church, Virginia, school system and conducts workshops for parents and kids throughout the area. She's a board member of SIECUS (Sex Information Education Council of the U.S.) and the Sex Education Coalition of Metropolitan Washington, among other organizations. You may have spotted her on some of your favorite TV talk shows. Ms. Tatum has two children.

Shirley Zussman, Ed.D., is a sex therapist with a nationwide reputation, whose opinion on matters of sexual functioning and sexual development is frequently sought by national publications. She is past president of AASECT and was co-director of the Long Island Jewish–Hillside Medical Center's Human Sexuality Center, which became one of the most prestigious sex therapy programs in the country. Dr. Zussman, a New Yorker, has two children. She lectures and publishes frequently: she is coauthor of *Getting Together, A Guide to Sexual Enrichment for Couples*.

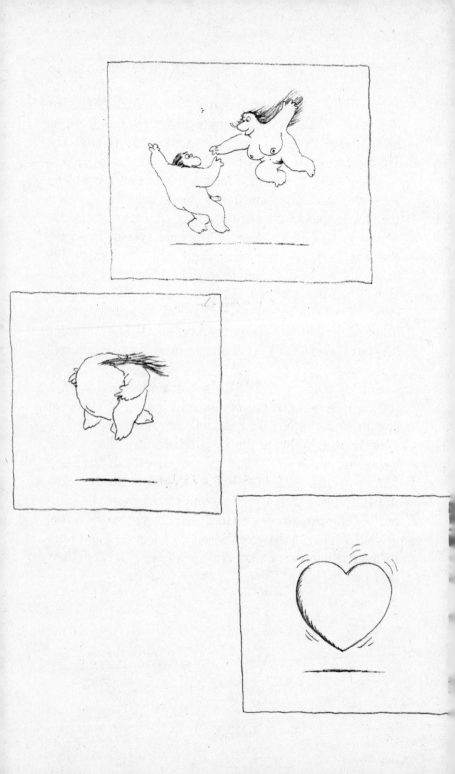

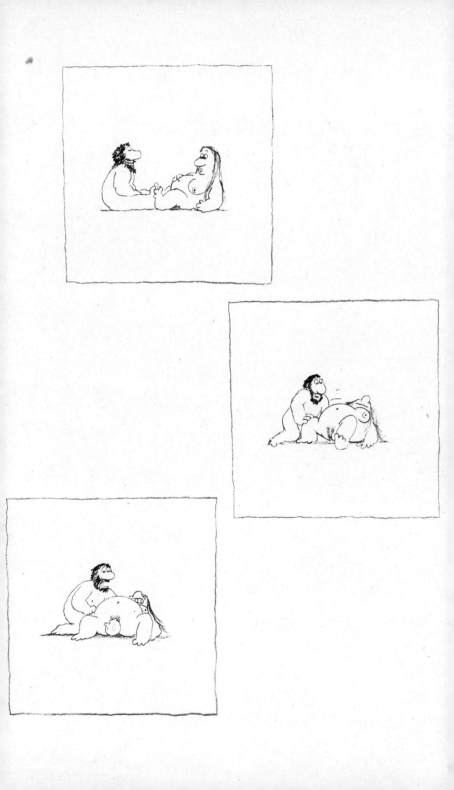

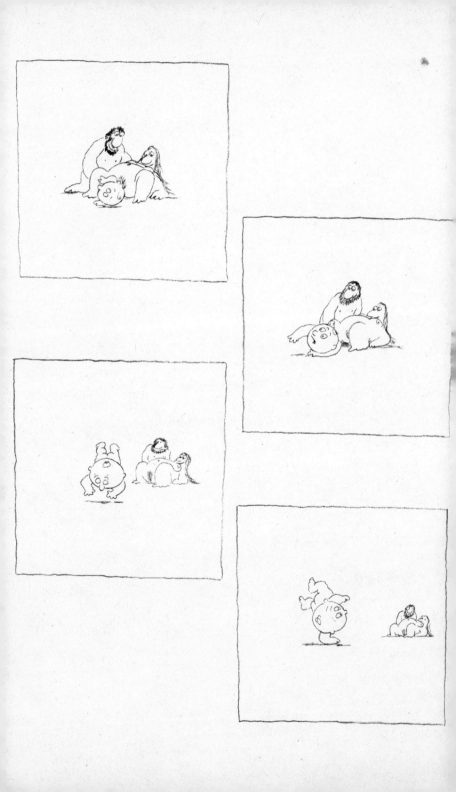

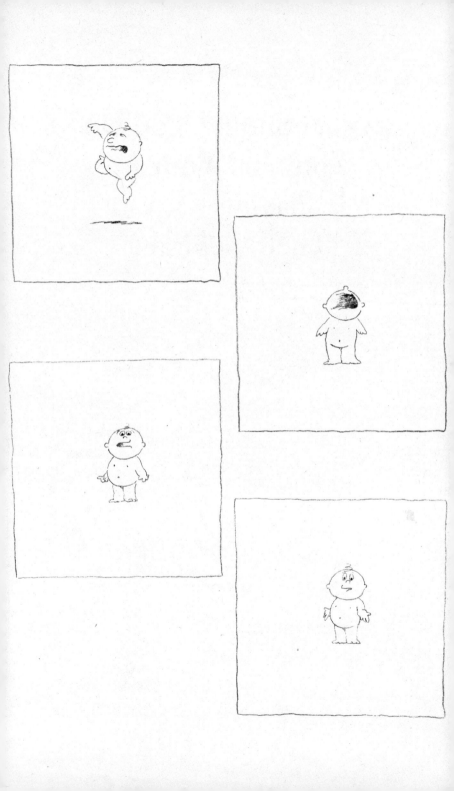

What Should You Do if You Find Your Kids Playing with Their Genitals?

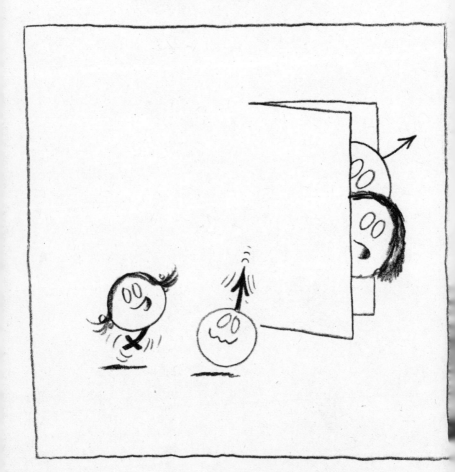

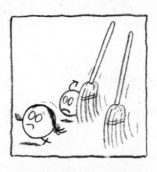

A. Stop them

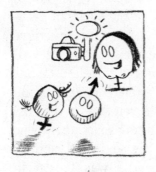

B. Encourage them

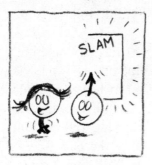

C. Ignore the situation

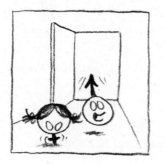

D. Accept the situation

Some days it all goes so easily. Being a parent seems the easiest and most rewarding job in the world. Truly, you have given life to a little angel who awakens with a smile, naps willingly, plays without complaint, returns to sleep with words of love on his sweet lips.

Other days are, well, more challenging. Today started out all right. The child woke up in a good mood, played by himself while you cleaned the house in preparation for your great-aunt, who was due to arrive for a week-long visit. After she came, he even allowed the elderly woman to hug, pinch, and kiss him. What a good boy! They seemed comfortable enough for you to leave them alone together while you saw to the casserole. When you returned to the living room, there was your little angel pulling on his little penis and smiling from ear to ear. Great-aunt Bertha was frozen in horror. Did she have a stroke? Why did he have to do this to you?

What are you going to do? Scream? Bribe him? Threaten him? Pretend that nothing in the world is going on—just tell Aunt Bertha that at her age people frequently see things? Or try being a "liberated" parent—mark this moment with a snapshot, the caption reading: "Markie discovers his penis the day Great-aunt Bertha arrives from Sioux City." Oh sure. Or you could plain and simply accept it. "Don't mind, Mark, Aunt Bertha, he's being a normal happy little boy." If you only had it in you.

Help! What's the Perfect Parent way to deal with this?

Most parents experience a lot of anxiety and mixed feelings over the question of their kids touching or playing with their genitals. They feel trapped somewhere between, "Oh oh, I'd better nip this nasty habit in the bud" and "What's the big deal?"

There is, however, no Perfect Parent answer—to this or to any other question of human sexuality. But there are, say the experts, a few things you *shouldn't* do. Like lose your cool.

"I think the best thing to do is to try to just be calm, cool, and collected," recommends Dr. Carol Cassell. "The worst thing to do is to utter the primitive scream." Such strong parental responses, she says, tend to become stuck in the kids' minds.

And reacting with shock and horror when you find your kids playing with themselves may convey some messages to them that you didn't really intend. First, the child may conclude that certain natural, pleasurable sensations of his or her body must be really bad if they can cause such reactions. It's an easy step from that conclusion to: anyone who has or wants to have these feelings must be pretty bad too.

Infants begin to explore their bodies within the first months of life—their feet, their hands, their ears, their genitals. Of course, when they happen upon their penises or clitorises, they discover feelings that may encourage them to linger a bit longer than at their elbows or their toes (which, especially to an infant, aren't half bad either). These discoveries are not only normal, they are important to the child's growth and development, ultimately playing a role in everything from self-acceptance to adult sexual response. It's tough to grow up feeling good about yourself if you can't feel good about certain parts of your anatomy and about how your body just naturally responds.

"I would like to see the day when a mother or father

walks in and finds little Suzy or Johnny touching themselves and can say, 'Oh, you've discovered how good that feels. Good for you!' " says Dr. Patricia Schreiner-Engel. "The point is that it's normal, it's natural, it's positive, and it's really helpful in terms of later adult sexual response."

The key word—for kids and parents too—is *natural*. Short of screaming bloody murder, what's the most natural response for you? Parents often want to stop their kids from touching themselves really because they feel embarrassed about seeing it. That's natural, because in our culture this is a private not a public behavior. If your kids are playing with themselves in the living room in front of Great-aunt Bertha or outside the home, you may feel more comfortable suggesting that they do it in their bedrooms, where they can close the door. Assure them that you won't disturb them. Privacy in itself is an important and special part of life, both for them and for you.

Some parents worry that once they make it okay for kids to play with themselves in their rooms that they'll never reemerge! But it's very rare, say the experts, that a child actually "overindulges."

Dr. Harold Lief: "Like any natural activity, there can, in rare instances, be an obsessive concern with it." This obsessive self-stimulation does *not* mean, he says, that your child is doing anything intrinsically harmful. What it may mean, though, is that the child is having a hard time coping with some personal or family troubles and needs your help to discover a more appropriate way to take the pressure off.

Like little Mark, having a fine time with himself out there in the living room, most kids are simply experiencing how nice it is to be alive. Sexuality is a part of life from the very beginning.

What Should You Do if You Find Your Kids Playing with Their Genitals?

    A. Stop them
    B. Encourage them
    C. Ignore the situation
  *D. **Accept the situation**

The experts agree that the best thing to do is to accept the situation, since it's perfectly natural—and utterly harmless.

Is It Harmful for Kids to See Their Parents Undressed?

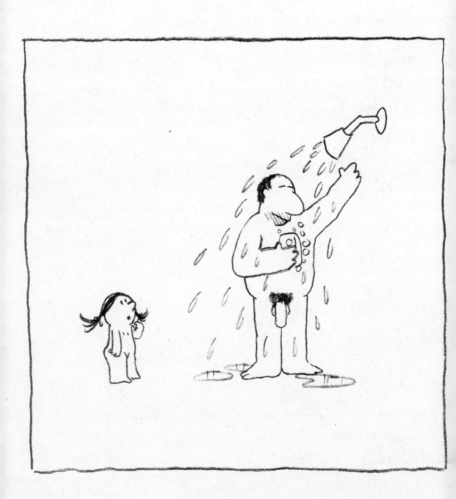

A. Yes

B. No

Should you trot around in the nude in front of your kids? This question is guaranteed to bring up a lot of strong feelings. Ask any four people:

"Oh no, absolutely not, never. Children should never see their parents undressed, not *totally*."

"I think that parents *should* walk around the house nude. Well, maybe not always. . . ."

"Baloney! The idea that nudity around the household is going to liberalize someone or make them more of a complete person went out with the sixties and the hippies. I'm a very complete adult man. My daughters aren't babies anymore. They're sixteen and fourteen. They're fairly complete themselves, if you know what I mean. I prefer to keep my clothes on around them. And I wish they'd keep them on in front of me."

"Why argue about it? It depends on who you are and what's right for you. Listen, my parents were adamant about me and my brother not coming in the bathroom or bedroom when they were undressed. So we both learned to knock and wait for an invitation." Speaking is a mother-to-be from Virginia named Linda. One day when Linda was about nine or ten her mother read a book that frightened her into believing that overly modest parents damage their kids' psyches. Linda didn't know that at the time, of course. When she knocked on her mother's door and she said to come in, Linda entered innocently—and found her mom standing stiff as a board in her birthday suit. Both of them just stood there awkward and embarrassed. Then Linda's father showed up, soon followed by her little brother, who was in turn followed by the family dog.

"It was winter and poor mom looked ice-cold. All of us stood and stared at her naked and shivering," Linda remembers. "Finally, my dad asked why in the world she was standing there like that, and mom mustered what little courage she had left and announced, 'Nudity is good, George.' He said, 'For whom?' But mom couldn't think of an answer to that. He handed her a robe and I escaped from the room."

Which of these four insistent opinions represents the experts' point of view?

They all do!

As Linda summed it up, it all depends on you. If you believe that parents should not be naked in front of their kids, then keep your clothes on. If you think that it's perfectly acceptable to be in your own house nude in front of your own children—you're right too. The point is, if you're comfortable being in your own home naked, fine. If you're not, don't worry about it. Do what's most comfortable; the right thing can't be right if it doesn't fit your style.

In any case, it is not going to hurt your child to see you without your clothes on. Children are naturally curious about their own bodies and about other people's bodies, yours included. What they see will contribute to their understanding of the human body and what to expect of their own bodies in years to come. If the parents are comfortable occasionally being without their clothes in the bathroom or in the bedroom when the kids are present, and if this has always been part of family life—nothing special or unusual, no showing off, nothing planned or manipulative—the message to the child is a positive one. It says: bodies are fine.

But if your birthday suit is not something you generally wear in front of other people, don't go tearing off your clothes because you think your children will benefit from your being less "uptight."

"It's unfortunate," comments Dr. Lyman Gilmore, "that if the parents read a book or feel guilty about not being more open about nudity in the home, and then experiment with being nude when they actually feel uncomfortable about it, all they end up conveying to the child is their own discomfort."

Be as open and comfortable with sexuality in your home as you can, say the experts—but be who you are. That's the most important thing.

More than the nudity itself, it's how you react to it—and how you react to your child when he or she accidentally catches you undressed—that most influences your kids. If your children have rarely seen you naked and one day burst in on you in the buff, the more upset you get, the more likely they are to remember your shocked reaction than what you looked like without your clothes on. They'll end up concluding that they must have done something bad, and that there's something bad about the naked body—conclusions that do not, in the long run, encourage a comfortable sexuality.

"Rather than acting as if a bomb has just been dropped," suggests Dr. Lief, simply "request your privacy."

"There's no great trauma over a child seeing a parent nude, opposite sex or same sex," reiterates Mary Lee Tatum. But to avoid a too-strong reaction on the parents' part, as well as possible confusion on the part of the child who has never seen his or her parents naked, most sex educators believe that families shouldn't worry too much about having to be fully dressed at all times when family members are together. Children who have seen an adult body from time to time have fewer misconceptions and fewer possibly upsetting surprises ahead of them.

Families in which nudity is more the rule than the exception needn't be concerned about "overexposure," because your kids will let you know when they think they've had enough. In early adolescence, when kids become more self-conscious about their own developing bodies, they'll retreat behind closed doors themselves and demand the same of you. In no uncertain terms they'll tell you: "Daddy, close your door!" and "Mommy, get out!" If that's what they want, say the educators and therapists, take the cue.

Is It Harmful for Kids to See
Their Parents Undressed?

A. Yes
*B. No

The experts agree that the answer is no. It isn't harmful for kids to see their parents undressed. But if you're not comfortable—or the child isn't—don't force it. Whatever feels right to you about nudity is probably going to be right for your kids too.

Question 3

How Early Should Parents Start Talking Sex with Their Kids?

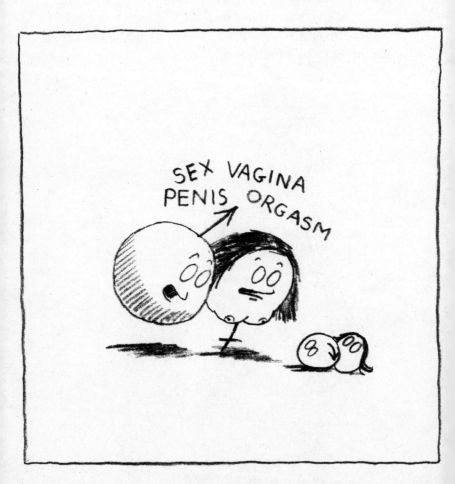

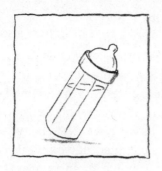

A. Infants

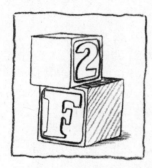

B. Toddlers

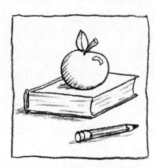

C. School age

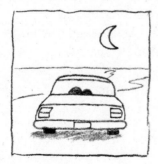

D. Teenagers

How old were you when your parents first mentioned the subject, if indeed they did? Most adults report that when they were adolescents their parents gave them some sort of talk or some advice, at least some hints about the propriety of sexual behavior. As everybody keeps saying, however, times have changed. If you wait till your kids are teenagers, you're liable to encounter something like this:

"John, you're getting to be quite a young man. I think it's time we had a little talk. You're old enough to know. Can you spare a few minutes? Oh, I see. You're late to pick up Jenny. Well, then, maybe we can speak when you get back later this evening. Oh, you're not coming back at all this evening? You're going to her folks' cabin for the whole weekend, are you? Her parents going to be there? No? Why, in my day. . . . Never mind, just um, hmm, be careful—I mean, drive carefully." And your sixteen-year-old pats you condescendingly on the shoulder and promises to have that talk with you when he gets back, as if he's going to teach *you* a thing or two. Which maybe he can.

But starting earlier has its own share of problems. Emily came home from first grade and asked her mother, "Mommy, where did I come from?"

Aha! just the moment I've been waiting for, thought Emily's modern mother, who launched into a well-rehearsed speech about penises and vaginas and sperms and uteruses. When she was through she asked the child what she thought about all this.

Emily shrugged. "Rachel says she came from Cincinnati and I was wondering where I came from."

Is there a right time?

Says Dr. Schreiner-Engel: "In order to help our children grow up to become happy, healthy adults, it's important for us as parents to start their 'sex education' when they are very, very young."

Even the first moments of their life is not too soon—once you understand what sex education really means. Most parents assume that sex education means telling the child "the facts of life" about intercourse, pregnancy, and birth—in other words, offering explanations about reproduction and all that goes along with it, including sexual feelings. But "sexual learning," as Mary Lee Tatum calls it, begins with the earliest awareness of ourselves and our bodies, other people and their bodies. Sexual attitudes begin to be shaped from birth by how a child is held and touched and loved and cared for and stimulated—and by how the parents hold, touch, love, and care for each other.

"Those natural things we do," says Ms. Tatum, "the hugging, kissing, touching, cuddling in families, are the best sex education we give our children."

The way in which the parents touch the children, the way in which they hold them, the way in which they touch each other, all convey the earliest messages about sexuality. And as soon as kids can understand the language, that's the time to begin talking about it.

Dr. Gilmore: "Probably the first words to the child about his or her body are really the beginning of sex education. Teaching the child that his or her body is a beautiful, God-given thing, that the penis and vagina are no more magical or forbidden than the nose or the ear, that bodies come in all sizes and shapes and colors, and that they're all okay—this gives a child a sense of well-being that is a foundation for a healthy sexuality in adolescence and adulthood."

Usually around the age of four or five, kids become curious not only about their own bodies, but about those of other people. "When they see differences between theirs and other bodies, they want to know why and how come," says Dr. Schreiner-Engel. "It's at that point that we as parents can effectively help them understand their bodies, to feel comfortable with them, and to understand and feel comfortable with themselves as male and female."

Sex educators believe that it is vitally important to give accurate information about all body parts and functions and to call them by their rightful names. Call a penis a penis. Describe to a little girl that she has a vulva which has many parts, including, among other things, a vagina and a clitoris. Parents who grew up in the "down-there" school, in homes where the genitals were mostly unmentionable, may find themselves at a loss for the correct vocabulary and may want to dash over to the local library (see the reading list at the end of this book).

What's wrong with good ol' "down there," "wee wee," "thing," and all those? For one, giving certain body parts cute or special names makes it seem that all body parts are not created equal. Some—like ears, or belly buttons—we can talk about in a perfectly straightforward way; but others, well, they're kind of um, ahem, embarrassing. The distinction goes a lot further than words, especially to kids: if you can't talk about something, there must be something wrong with it.

And not using the real words can make it pretty

tough to communicate. "Kindergarten teachers often talk about the terrible problem they have that each family has a different pet name for the different parts of the anatomy, which becomes difficult for kids as they get in with other kids," says Dr. Cassell. One has a peter, another a ding-dong, another a ti-ti—and nary a penis or vagina in the room!

Not to mention confusion. How many kids who have been told that daddy puts his seed into mommy's tummy go through childhood believing that sex is a quasi-agricultural/digestive function?

The kind of information kids seek and what they can understand change as they grow up, beginning with their little body-universes in which all reality seems to be centered. From the start, educators advise, keep your explanations straightforward and honest, and keep the story the same. Instead of having daddy starting a garden in mommy's stomach, have penis-vagina-uterus-egg-sperm in the repertoire from the beginning, and elaborate with more sophisticated details as your children mature. This way you'll be providing your kids with a solid, consistent foundation on which their sexuality and their understanding can slowly and appropriately unfold.

But as always with kids—little ones, big ones, even grown-up ones—actions speak louder than words. "Really, what's more important than talking about sex with kids is the way parents act with each other," says Dr. Lief. "Kids learn so much by watching their parents interact, the exchange of affection, those little pats of tenderness."

Sexuality is, after all, something that's expressed so much of the time just by how we look at the other person, how we touch each other, how we carry our bodies, how we smile and laugh. Kids learn a lot, perhaps most, from what they see and feel around them. That starts the first day of their lives.

How Early Should Parents Start Talking Sex with Their Kids?

*A. **Infants**
 B. Toddlers
 C. School age
 D. Teenagers

Surprisingly, the experts tell us that kids begin to learn about sex in infancy—by the way they're held, by the way they're touched, and by the relationships they see around them. So even before they can talk, your kids are learning about sex and their own bodies.

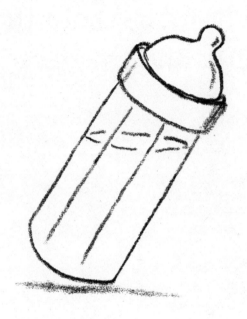

Can You Tell Your Kids Too Much About the Birds and the Bees?

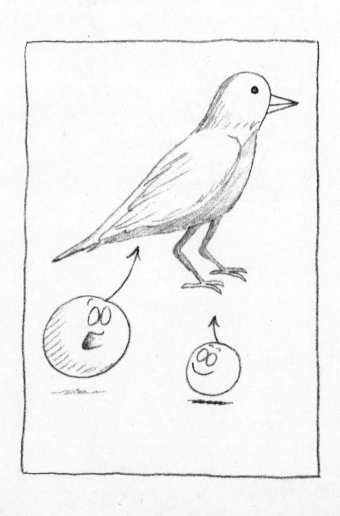

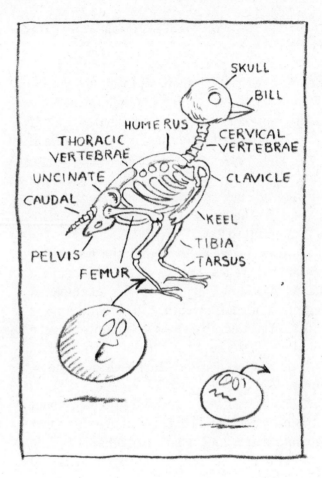

A. Yes

B. No

If you tell your kids that not only do penises go inside vaginas, but that what happens next is as good as—no, better than—candy, pizza, potato chips, and ice cream . . . will they start going in for new afterschool treats?

If you tell your teenage daughter about birth control, will her boyfriend be the first to thank you?

Do they have to know *everything*? Can kids learn too much too fast? If you tell them all the juicy details, won't they want to go out and try for themselves?

"A lot of parents and teachers are worried that if you talk to children about sexuality, it's going to lead them to be sexual. They are concerned that sex education causes sexual exploration or sexual curiosity or sexual promiscuity," acknowledges Dr. Gilmore. "That just isn't true. We don't have any evidence that information is harmful to kids."

There's more evidence, in fact, that the *less* information a child has, the less able he or she is to make a wise decision regarding sex, when, for example, a friend suggests a sexual adventure. The child who is informed is less vulnerable to the misinformation about sex and about the results of sexual activity than is the child who has learned the "facts" through hearsay and innuendo.

Similarly, the more growing children know about how good the body feels or is capable of feeling, what sex and sexuality are, and what really happens, the better they tend to behave in adolescence, when sexual activity earnestly begins.

"My experience is that kids who do not feel good about their bodies do not feel good about sex, and they make bad decisions about the way in which they relate to each other sexually," says Mary Lee Tatum. There is some evidence, she says, that in families in which there is open communication about sex (and everything else), kids tend to wait before they have sexual intercourse—welcome news for parents who worry that if they give their kids the full scoop on the birds and the bees they'll go right out and do it.

Besides, giving information to kids, as educator Tatum puts it, "is like taking vitamins—their body uses what it needs and gets rid of the rest. Children are focused on one aspect of the answer. As soon as they have that," she says, "they want to know whether they can go out and play or if they can have another piece of French toast."

Adds Dr. Cassell, "Kids are great at turning parents off. Just test this out by trying to explain to them why they should take care of their rooms and clean up. Watch their eyes glaze over. They do the same thing about sex. They turn off things that they don't want to hear about. They are, of course, curious about sex and probably a little more interested in that than in cleaning their room, but, truly, there is nothing to fear. You can't tell a kid too much or too soon."

What the kids will hear of what you tell them will change as they grow and develop. All the more reason to keep telling the sex story over and over and over as the years go by. A toddler who wants to know about sex may really be interested only in the difference between males and females and not listen to how babies are made. A child of ten or eleven may find descriptions of penises entering vaginas utterly tedious and would rather know why anybody would *want* to do this. Older children are curious about feelings, responses, relationships and will absorb these details most readily.

While there's little chance you'll turn your kids into sex maniacs by giving them all the information they crave, there *is* a chance you'll bore them to tears. Sex educators agree that if information is thrown at a kid in a dry, cold, pedantic, unfeeling way, the child may avoid talking about sex with you and will turn instead to other sources—like other kids.

The best way to avoid turning them off is not to talk over their heads and to remember that sex and sexuality is not all physiology. Respond at their level. How do you know what that is? Dr. Schreiner-Engel offers a good way to figure this out:

"Let's say a child asks you how come his penis gets so large or where do babies come from; these are classic questions. To find out how to respond, say, 'That's a good question,' and ask him what *he* thinks the answer to the question is. Then you can start either at the level of his real knowledge or at the point where he becomes confused or possesses misinformation. This technique will help you to target right in to the kind of knowledge that the child needs to know at that point."

This technique also works with older children. When her eleven-year-old daughter kept asking how exactly a woman goes about having sex, a Providence, Rhode Island, mother repeatedly explained that the woman spreads her legs and the man puts his penis in her vagina. But her daughter never seemed satisfied with the answer. A week or two would go by and she'd ask again. Finally the woman asked the child how she thought women did it.

"First the woman takes off all her clothes," the girl said shyly. "Then she stands on her head, then she spreads her legs, then . . ."

"Of course I stopped her," says the girl's mother. "I asked her why she thought the woman had to stand on her head. She said her friend Suzie swore it was true. Apparently it had really been bothering her and that's why she kept asking me. She had all the other facts right, after my numerous explanations. But I had never explained how it was possible to do it while standing on your head. She was worried she'd never get it right. She said she almost managed a headstand once in gym class, but then she tried to spread her legs and she fell right over."

Can You Tell Your Kids Too Much About the Birds and the Bees?

A. Yes
*B. No

It seems that when it comes to sex, kids take in information at their own speed. Since they'll take in only as much as they can handle, you don't have to worry about telling your kids too much about sex. And there will always be more they need to know.

Between Parent and Child, What's Off-Limits?

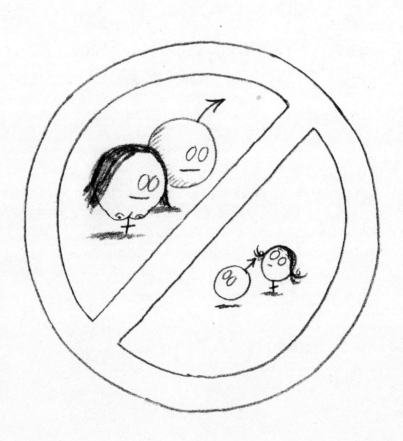

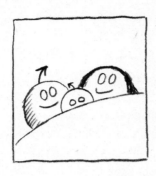

A. Snuggling in bed with parents

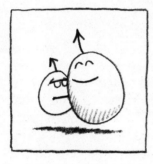

B. Father-son embraces

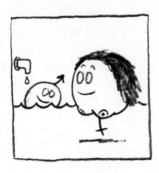

C. Mothers bathing sons

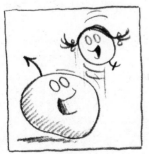

D. Father-daughter roughhousing

E. None of the above

Sharing affection in families can be the greatest. Hugging and holding bring us close. But is there such a thing as too close? Frank, Jr., always climbs into bed with his parents on Sunday mornings. He brings them the big weekend paper, hands each of them a section, and warmly nestles in-between them. But Frank's mother is beginning to wonder whether she should put a stop to it. Frank is, after all, forty-four, and his father has begun to get upset—he says Junior always hogs the Sports section.

Bathe Frank? Good gracious no, his mother laughs. Why, she hasn't done that since he was eighteen. . . .

Where should you draw the line? Parents worry that some situations involving close bodily contact with their children may have sexual overtones. When it comes to your kids snuggling in bed with you, for example, is there some magic age, short of forty-four, when suddenly things change and it would be better for them—and for you—if they'd keep out?

The answer to that is: no, there is no magic age and there are no hard-and-fast rules. Within families, the natural and spontaneous intimacies—touching and being close, hugging and snuggling—when you are in bed or out, are moments to be treasured by parents and children alike. Just keep an eye out, say the experts, for when the pattern of affection and needs for closeness seem to change.

If snuggling in bed together has never been your family's way and now all of a sudden your child is perpetually requesting to climb in, or if you find yourself wanting the kids there to hug and to cuddle more than before, you might ask yourself: what is going on here? What is going on in your or your child's life that might account for the neediness? If you can figure out what it is, then you can decide whether physical intimacy is the best way to respond.

The key question for parents is not what you "should" or "shouldn't" do at any given time, but, as Dr. Gilmore says, "Whose needs are being met?" Sometimes, he says, in families in which there has been a death or a separation or a divorce, without realizing it the remaining parent, out of loneliness and neediness, begins to seek more intimacy from the children. "This isn't so much a sexual gratification as a kind of 'loneliness gratification,'" he explains. Nevertheless, it could put too much pressure on the kids, which might lead to some difficulties.

In most situations, though, Dr. Gilmore stresses, "by far it's much more important to be close and to be intimate and to be touching with children and to enjoy physical intimacy with them—if that's what you feel comfortable with." Don't do it, though, because you think it's "right" or you think you "should." But if it *feels* right—sure!

Speaking of comfortable, in many families a father may feel natural and happy embracing and kissing his baby son, but as the boy grows older, dad may begin to wonder whether he shouldn't cut this physical stuff out. He begins to distance himself from his son and to show his affection for him from arm's length. So what used to be a hug and a kiss becomes a cool pat on the shoulder or a handshake. This, many fathers believe, is more masculine.

But are father-son embraces inappropriate?

Dr. Lief: "There's nothing wrong whatsoever with a father and son embracing. Our culture is really hung up about being macho. Supposedly it's not 'masculine' to embrace or kiss another male," although other cultures, such as the French, don't seem to worry so much about it, he points out. "So natural affection between fathers and sons, between brothers, between friends, is often avoided because of this false societal myth and taboo."

This myth often deprives boys of the closeness of their fathers just when they need it most, at the onset of adolescence. Enduring such intense conflict and confusion, they need to be hugged and held and reassured more than ever before . . . although they may not act as if they do.

"Something happened to me a number of years ago that still brings a little choke to my throat," recalls Dr. Gilmore. He was leaving his home in New Hampshire for six weeks in order to conduct some postdoctoral research in Ohio. Never had he been away from his family for so long a time. "I remember my wife and my daughter and my son were lined up on the back porch of our house. I gave my wife a big hug and a kiss, I gave my daughter a big hug and a kiss, and I shook my son's hand."

Only after he had left did it strike Dr. Gilmore that just as his father had stopped hugging and kissing him when he was a young adolescent, "I had stopped doing it with my own son." And now he wouldn't even see his son for another six weeks. "It was a moving lesson for me that perhaps I should reach out to him, as my father did not reach out to me when I was a child." Subsequently, Dr. Gilmore did reach out to his son, and ultimately to his father too. ("My father is eighty-

WHAT'S OFF-LIMITS? • 49

one," he says, "and we've developed a new kind of intimacy. We hug each other whenever we see each other. That's been beautiful for him and it's been beautiful for me.")

Fathers and sons (not to mention the family females), it seems, all need their share of physical closeness. "One of the biggest hungers adults have is to be touched," Dr. Schreiner-Engel tells us, and this need continues through our lives to our very oldest years.

No one would question mothers and daughters hugging and kissing, and it is usually not considered off-limits for moms to hold and hug their teenage sons. In our culture this seems perfectly natural. But mama bathing her "baby" six-footer—that's another story.

When it comes to mothers bathing sons, sex educators agree that there's a point at which mom ought to retire from bathtub duty and let junior do the work himself. The issue here is encouraging kids to take care of themselves and be independent, and thus the advice to mom to step out holds for her and her daughter as well.

When are kids old enough to bathe themselves? For most kids, that's about the time they start school. You still may want to run the water for them and make sure there's soap, and you'll want to check up on the little ones from time to time. But don't spend too much time trying to gauge the perfectly "right" moment to hand over the soap, because chances are the kids will tell you. As kids grow up they begin to want their privacy—they'll want you out of the bathroom and the door shut. "That's the time when mothers have to stop bathing sons," says Dr. Carol Cassell, "when they develop a sense of privacy." Always respect and support their desire for privacy, the experts advise, and teach them to respect yours, too.

What about fathers and daughters roughhousing? Is there a point at which Dad should keep his hands off? This is a tough question for some dads, who, as their daughters develop breasts and figures, naturally find them kind of sexy. Knowing that they find their daughters attractive, they wonder whether touching them and horsing around the way they always used to now has sexual connotations.

It is appropriate, of course, for a father to examine his behavior and decide what his motivations and reactions really are. If his daughter's approaching womanhood does make him—or her—jumpy when they have physical contact, then for both their sakes he ought to change his style. But that doesn't mean that fathers should stop being physically close to their daughters. As Dr. Shirley Zussman points out, "There are plenty of ways besides roughhousing, if need be, to having some physical involvement. You can put your arm around her. You can hold her hand and go for a walk."

Like adolescent boys, girls need physical closeness with their fathers, for the same and for different reasons. During these critical years of maturing sexuality, girls need to maintain "their sense of being touchable and that their body is a good thing, and they need to know, too, that they are allowed to touch their father," says Dr. Patricia Schreiner-Engel. "This kind of affectional touching is extremely important psychologically." If, as her body begins to change, dad gets nervous and sets up a no-touch barrier between him and his not-so-little girl, she's liable to draw some unfortunate conclusions about her sexuality—that her maturing body can't be all that good if it drove her dad away.

So, say the experts, fathers should try to keep tuned in to how both they and their daughters are feeling. If both of you seem comfortable with the same old roughhousing you've always engaged in, there's no reason to have to stop completely. But find some other ways to stay close if it just doesn't feel right anymore.

Between Parent and Child, What's Off-Limits?

A. Snuggling in bed with parents
B. Father-son embraces
C. Mothers bathing sons
D. Father-daughter roughhousing
*E. **None of the above**

The answer is that none of these is necessarily off-limits. But the answer is complicated. Kids need affection, but they also need independence. As kids get older, some things are no longer appropriate. And for some parents, some behaviors just aren't comfortable anymore.

Is It Harmful if Your Child Accidentally Catches You in the Act?

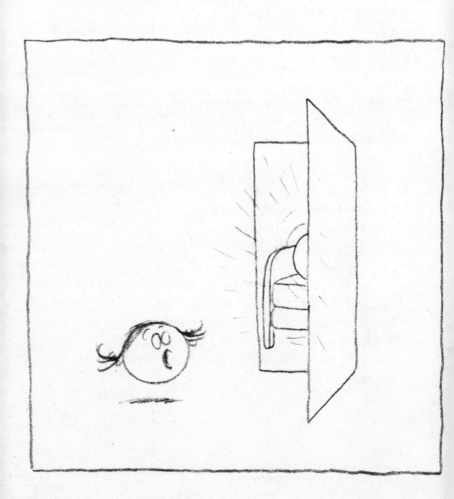

A. Yes

B. No

Fortunately, when you were a child, this wasn't a problem. Your parents didn't have sex. Unthinkable! They did it to make their babies and then they stopped.

Now that you are a parent, though, you are willing to grant that maybe, just maybe, they did "it" too. But how did they manage it utterly without notice? You don't remember hearing beds creaking, or peculiar noises coming from their room. Not once did your parents sound like they didn't want you to come in when you needed them in the middle of the night (well, there was that one time . . .). Did your daddy sneak back in the house after you and your brother and sister had gone to school? Did they wait until three o'clock in the morning (in high school your older sister was notorious for staying up reading romance novels until two). It's possible they waited until they went away on vacation. But that happened only every three or four years.

One day curiosity gets the best of you. You ask your father how he and your mom managed to be so quiet about their lovemaking. He looks up in shock from his ham sandwich. "What kind of question is that?" And says no more.

Well then, maybe they didn't do it. You've had the impression for some time anyway that sex was invented in the 1960s.

And along with sex came paper-thin walls, floors that could cause the whole house to sway in a certain rhythm, doors that won't stay closed, and paralyzing anxiety that the kids are going to catch you at it.

Some parents worry so much about the consequences that they can't comfortably make love when the kids are anywhere in the house. But it's the parents who are more likely to suffer from the interruption (if not the inhibition), say the experts, than the kids are from the unexpected eyeful.

"I would have been horrified if either of our kids had walked in on us when we were making love," Dr. Lyman Gilmore admits, "but I don't think kids are horrified. I've talked to many young people about this kind of thing and they giggle and laugh and say 'Gross!' "

But when they don't know what's going on—and little kids usually haven't a clue what it is you're doing —it's important to explain, so that they don't come to some upsetting conclusions. "Intercourse has a semi-violent look to it to young kids," says Dr. Cassell. "And since in many homes kids don't see their parents nude, that can also be a shock."

Tell your child that this is what grown-ups do when they want to show their love. Let them know that it is something that feels good, even though it may look like daddy was trying to hurt mommy. Depending on the age of the child, you might want to mention that this is the way that babies are made. Noises, too, can scare a child; point out that the sounds mean that you really like what you are doing, even though they might sound like you're uncomfortable.

You needn't do all this talking instantly; no doubt you have other things on your mind. However, "If the child appears disturbed by it, try to give him or her some kind of reassurance and explanation at that moment," suggests Dr. Zussman. "If the child is half-asleep, I'd wait until the next morning."

Whatever you do, don't panic and overreact. "The response of the parent is crucial and becomes the message that the child carries away from the experience. Any kind of violent response will further confuse the child and contribute to a kind of ambivalence about sex," says Dr. Gilmore.

An ounce of prevention is worth a pound of cure. Mary Lee Tatum advises: "Calmly tell them, 'This is the way we show each other that we love each other'—then put a lock on the door." Why worry about being interrupted every time you make love? Kids can appreciate privacy if you tell them about it, as long as they know they can knock if they need you.

Although parents are advised to try to create an atmosphere of quiet and privacy for their own sakes as well as for the sake of the child, it's doubtful whether you'll always be able to conceal the fact that you are making love. "Kids know when their parents are having sex," says Dr. Gilmore. "The very act of being careful creates a special condition in the house and the kids know something's up." In families where sex is an open and comfortable subject, where kids are encouraged to understand that sex exists, where doors lock, why worry?

Kids' awareness does get a little more complicated in single-parent households. It won't hurt them to know that there's such a thing as intercourse, but it takes some additional discussion when sex partners tend to change. "Kids don't think, 'Oh, isn't mommy or daddy having a wonderful time and I'm so glad,' " Mary Lee Tatum points out. They may feel very jealous.

So talk it out. In whatever language is appropriate to the age of your kids, let them know that you care for your partner and that you are going to be in the bedroom together, where you will be expressing love the way adults do. "Then give the children an opportunity to vent whatever emotions that they may be feeling," says Dr. Gilmore. "Reward them for doing that, because kids need to do that to take care of themselves."

It's usually easiest for kids to deal with sex-and-the-single-parent if you wait until your relationship is on a solid footing before you bring someone new into your home for the night, say the therapists.

In the long run, your kids will appreciate being sure their parents had (and still have) a sex life. It's something that doesn't involve them, that's for sure. But if they know, that's life!

Is It Harmful if Your Child Accidentally Catches You in the Act?

A. Yes
*B. No

Sex educators and therapists are no longer concerned that kids will be traumatized if they accidentally barge in while their parents are making love. But kids can come to some pretty funny conclusions about the meaning of such a peculiar-looking activity. So be sure they understand that although this is something that parents do in the strictest privacy, it's a really nice thing.

Question 7

Where Do Most Kids Find Out About Sex?

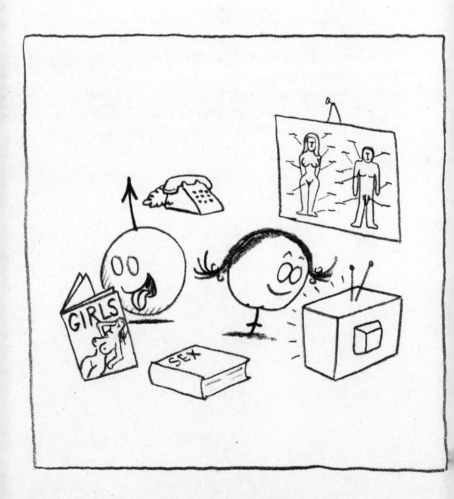

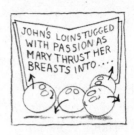

A. Magazines and books

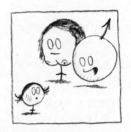

B. Parents

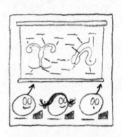

C. Sex-education programs

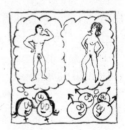

D. Friends

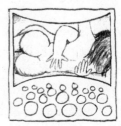

E. TV and movies

You were once a kid yourself. Do you remember where you first found out about sex?

"Dirty jokes in the back seat of the school bus."

"From my older brother's collection of dirty books."

"Our science teacher told us. But I thought he must be joking around. He sure had a sick sense of humor. I mean, if that stuff were true, I was sure my mom would have told me about it."

"From books my mom would leave on my shelf. She'd say, 'Don't you think it's about time you cleaned your bookcases?' and that's how I'd know there was a new sex book waiting for me. So I'd read it; then my best friend Judy would explain what it *really* meant. That's how I learned that a man and a woman do IT only once, and the man leaves as many sperm as he's got, from one to maybe six or seven, inside her. Then the woman proceeds to have as many babies as the number of sperm. You see, she never knew how many she'd end up having. Which explained why some kids had a lot of brothers and sisters and I had none."

"I learned from other boys. My father had one talk with me when I was seventeen. He gripped the wheel of the car and mumbled something—I knew it was important because he was mumbling. Something about, 'Girls . . . mumble, mumble . . . don't. . . .' "

"I learned about sex by just doing it."

"Sex? What's sex?"

Kids today seem to know an awful lot more about sex than we did. They can't avoid it. It's all over TV, in the movies, on the magazine and book racks in the corner drugstore, in advertisements; they even see it exhibited in the flesh on city streets. And the new openness about sexual matters has begun to encourage sex-education programs in schools and greater communication with parents.

Among all sources, where are kids today most likely to learn about sex?

From each other, same as we did.

According to some accounts, the kiddie sex grapevine is even more active now than it used to be. As early as the second grade it's abuzz with all the "facts" that our present-day society exposes kids to. The problem is, our children are no more capable of understanding it all or putting it in the correct context than we were. Kids are kids; it takes them a long time to comprehend the complexities of life. Kids today end up having an enormous vocabulary of sex, which they don't necessarily comprehend, especially if their parents aren't explaining and interpreting it all for them.

So with all the information they have to give to one another, and they certainly have a lot, kids today are passing around even more *mis*information than we did.

Some of the false information kids pass on to each other is cute. ("When a man and a woman do it, the man puts his thing through a hole in the woman's nightgown." "My mommy doesn't have holes in her nightgowns." "Mine doesn't either. That's how I know they don't do it.") Most often, though, misinformation is damaging, says Mary Lee Tatum. "For instance, some boys in the fifth, sixth, and seventh grades may get hold of the false information that if they masturbate they are homosexual. That sets up a terrible anxiety at a very early age, when a child isn't ready to deal with it. That myth should be dispelled by adults," she says emphatically.

What kids need—and, as it turns out, what they *want*—is for their parents to explain what all this sex stuff means. They need help making sense of it in terms of their own lives and experiences, and to help them to understand what is ahead for them as boys and girls, men and women, physically and emotionally.

"A vast majority of kids say that they did not get adequate information about sexuality at home, and all of them wish they had," reports Dr. Lyman Gilmore. "That's really the place where it can be done. Parents clearly are the normal, natural source of information about sexuality—yet kids don't get it from them."

A lot of parents feel funny bringing up the subject out of nowhere ("So, um, tell me son, cough cough, how's the old masturbating going?") Thinking it'll be easier on everybody if they just wait for the children to ask questions, parents may create an atmosphere of silence that says to the child: We don't talk about that here. So the child who has important questions about sex—and virtually every child has—will turn to a friend for "wisdom," or try to reason it him- or herself, often resulting in erroneous conclusions about sex or about themselves that may influence the course of smooth sexual development.

Don't think, though, that when kids confide to sex educators that they wish their parents would talk about sex with them that all they want to hear is the mechanical stuff—insert part A into part B, etc. Even if they learn the physiological aspects in school, they still wish their parents would contribute their side of things.

Reveals Dr. Cassell: "They'd love to have their parents talk to them about love. They want to know whether their parents are in love, what love is like. They're very interested in knowing how their parents met, and parents frequently fluff over information like that. But, especially, kids want to know from parents what they think about love."

They want to know what love feels like, what it means, how to know if another person is in love with you. Understanding and acceptance of love and a desire to love are at the basis of a person's sexuality. For the parents who bemoan our society's tendency to separate sex from love, here's a golden opportunity to do a little gluing.

And kids are dying to know what "sexy" means. What is a boy "supposed" to be like to be attractive? What "should" a girl look like or do? Kids get contradictory and, unfortunately, powerful impressions about that from advertisements, magazines, TV, movies. But what do their parents believe?

If you can talk to your kids about sex and the full range of sexuality, then they know they can talk to you about it. They can bring their questions and confusions to you and not rely on the wisdom of the self-proclaimed expert in the playground. When they are making decisions about their own sexual behavior, with a history of open sexual discussion in the family, they may trust you enough to ask for your help.

Remember, kids are not so sophisticated about sex

as we might think these days. If you listen closely, you will notice that rock lyrics convey one explicit sex message after another. A father of a six-year-old was horrified to hear his daughter and a male friend going around singing "let's get physical, let's get physical. . . ." Finally he could restrain himself no longer and insisted she stop singing such a song—she was just plain too young to be involved with such a notion. But for the life of her, she couldn't figure out what was wrong with what she was singing.

"Don't you know what 'let's get physical' means?" asked the exasperated father.

"Sure," she replied. "It's like, you know, getting"— she searched for the word—"athletic. Playing tennis and riding your bike, going swimming, playing basketball and baseball, jogging. . . ." [Boy, sometimes dads are really dumb.]

Where Do Most Kids Find Out About Sex?

    A. Magazines and books
    B. Parents
    C. Sex-education programs
 *D. Friends
    E. TV and movies

It turns out that most of today's kids are still learning about sex from other kids—but they'd really like to learn about it from their parents. They are not interested only in the facts of life, though. They want to know about the feelings of love. So even if your kids have never asked you about sex, don't think that they're not interested or that they don't need the kind of information only you can give them.

What Should You Do if Your Kids Use Dirty Words?

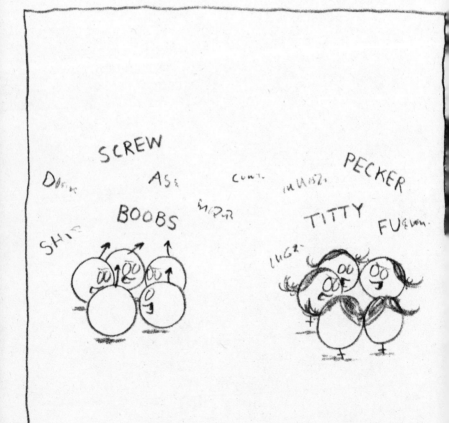

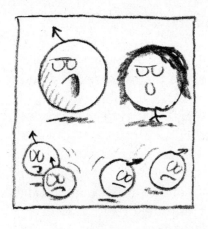 **A.** Forbid it

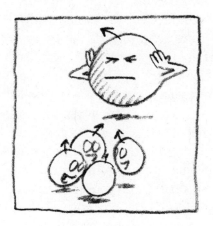 **B.** Close your ears

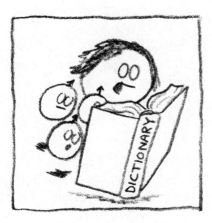 **C.** Explain what the words mean

Some families handle this little problem very creatively. One family made a rule that whoever uttered a curse word or a dirty word, adult or child, would have to deposit twenty-five cents into a kitty. The idea backfired. At the end of the year, the kitty was so fat that mom, dad, and three kids ages seven to fifteen could spend their "earnings" at the fanciest restaurant in town. The next year they abandoned the penalties and the tone of their language improved considerably.

Another family, with two boys ages eight and thirteen, held several family conferences to decide which words were okay, which were definitely off-limits, and which were in a gray area in between. They studied each word and its variations very carefully. They decided, as one example, that you could never say "bullshit," you could say "b.s." around the house if you absolutely had to, but you could say nothing at all around grandmother (that gray area). "Fuck" was always off-limits, but if you were feeling seriously hostile and had to get the feeling off your chest, you could raise four fingers (never one) to indicate that a four-letter word was strongly on your mind.

Still another family attempted a geographical solution. Certain words you could mutter to yourself in the privacy of your room if you absolutely had to. Other words could come as far as the living room, depending on who was in it, but none of these words were to enter the dining room. Some were okay in the lobby of the building but not in the elevator if non-family members were in it. Some were okay in the playground but never in the classroom. One of the kids, age thirteen, got it into her bright mind to draw a map that portrayed all the geographical possibilities. The problem was that there wasn't a room in the house in which she was allowed to hang it, with all those shocking words.

There's always the good old-fashioned solution: "If you say that again I'll wash your mouth out with soap." But has anyone figured out how you go about doing that? Do you use bar soap or soapsuds?

One thing's for sure: Kids do love dirty and racy words and parents do *not* like them to be used. Parental reactions range from annoyance to serious moral indignation. But even if you include yourself in the latter category, try not to make a big issue out of it when the little darling drops the first profane bombshell. The reason is a practical one. Your angry reaction will reinforce the power of that word to get a rise out of you. Kids, even little ones, usually know there's something racy or wrong about dirty words, and they often test their parents with them, "using them as a string to make mommy jump," says Mary Lee Tatum.

"Take it seriously," says Ms. Tatum, "but don't make a huge issue out of it. Go on making your chocolate-chip cookies," and while you do, quietly explore where the child heard the word (and be prepared that he or she may have gotten it from you). Then ask the child whether he or she knows what it means. If not, explain in a simple way that the child can understand. Explain too why you do not want this word or this kind of language to be used.

"If the parent finds this kind of word very upsetting, I think it's okay for the parent to say, 'I don't like that word and I would rather you didn't say it,' " says Dr. Shirley Zussman. "It really has to do with the comfort of the parent."

Your kids will learn soon enough that there's a wide variance in the acceptability of slang words from household to household, sometimes between adults and children in the same household. Culturally, the use of off-color language is not as "damnable" as it used to be, although prohibitions vary from group to group and may depend on the particular social circumstance —all quite complicated and difficult to explain to a child. Begin by letting your kids know what it is about these words that makes *you* so uncomfortable; then set clear limits on what's acceptable in your household.

"Do you have a religious conviction that this word is morally damaging to your child?" asks Dr. Carol Cassell. "Or do you find it simply offensive? Perhaps you feel that the language is abusive or hostile or violent. Or maybe you feel that it's not 'nice.' Or the bottom line may be that in your circle it is not socially acceptable."

You may not be awfully upset by a word, may indeed use it yourself, but still not wish your child to use it, at least not in his or her "everyday" vocabulary or outside the house. Then your challenge will be to help the child develop discrimination. Dr. Zussman notes: "You might say, 'Some people use those words, but other people are bothered by them. Maybe if you need to say those words or want to say them, say them here or say them to yourself or to your friend if your friend knows them. But it's not the kind of word you use in class or when you're visiting.' Do try to differentiate that there are times that it's okay and times it's not, and that some people don't want to hear them at any time.

"And if the child says, 'Look, you use this word yourself,' you can point out, 'True, but I don't do it on my job or at the table. I just say it when I'm very, very angry.' "

"Talk about the consequences," Dr. Gilmore suggests. "Depending on the age of the child, you can say, for instance, 'Do you want to make grandma unhappy? No? Well, that's one of the words we don't say in front of grandma because, for reasons that are pretty complicated, we don't say certain words at certain times. They make some people unhappy or embarrassed. And if you say these words in front of a teacher, you'll get in trouble.'"

Outside of the varying social, religious, and cultural consequences, the principal objection that most sex educators and therapists have to kids' using this language is what it has to say about sex. Most "dirty" sexual words are associated with anger, hostility, and aggression, particularly in the relation of the male to the female.

"The real problem with dirty words is that they denigrate something that most people consider to be a transcendent spiritual experience," says Dr. Gilmore. To use a word like "fuck" for making love, he says, "is really creating an attitude about sexuality that equates it with dirtiness and forbiddenness and animalism. For a fifteen-year-old who is confused or simply inexperienced, thinking about sex in these terms creates a nastiness about it that may never be overcome."

Dirty words do serve one useful purpose, however. "They keep us from hitting each other over the head with rocks," explains Dr. Gilmore. Civilized people have to find a way to express hostility and rage short of physically attacking one another. So we hurl taboo words and epithets. And kids learn to toss a few themselves. It's too bad, though, that so many of our insults have to do with sex.

What Should You Do if Your Kids Use Dirty Words?

   A. Forbid it
   B. Close your ears
*C. **Explain what the words mean**

Sexual slang is widely used in today's society. But dirty words mean different things to different people. Kids won't know what they mean to you unless you explain it to them.

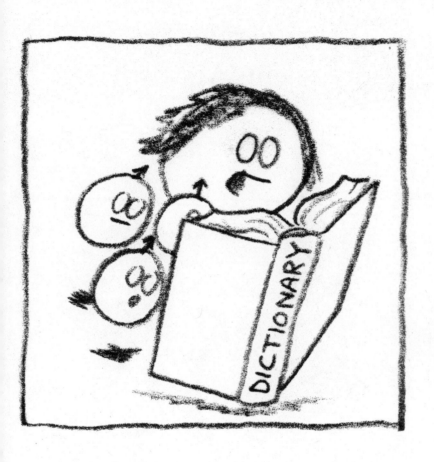

What Percentage of Adolescents Masturbate?

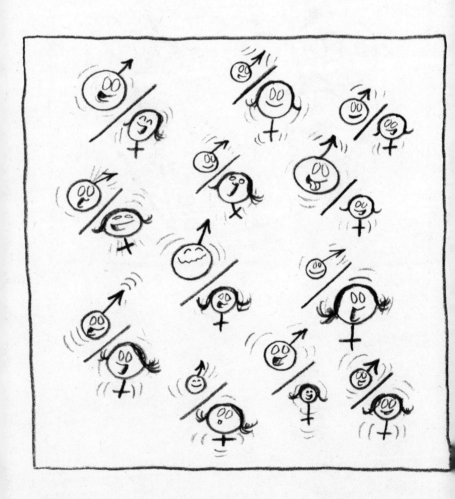

Before we get to this question, let us take a quick run down memory lane and review some of the favorite old masturbation myths. Which one terrorized *you* most when you were a child?

Masturbation drains your brains, makes you crazy, turns your gray matter to slush.

Keep it up and it will cripple you.

If you masturbate you will become homosexual.

If you masturbate hair will grow on the palm of your hand. And it will fall out from the top of your head.

Your penis will get shorter. It will fall off.

Your vagina will shrivel. It will close up.

Your hands will fall off.

Your thumbs will fall off.

You'll get infected.

You'll smell.

You'll turn into a boy.

You'll turn into a girl.

You'll turn into a pervert.

You already are a pervert.

Masturbation makes you introverted.

If you masturbate you will never enjoy a *real* orgasm.

If you masturbate you'll get hooked on yourself and lose interest in having sex with another person. Or the other person will lose interest in having sex, or anything else, with you.

Your toes will fall off.

You'll get a rash.

You'll get pimples. Really disgusting ones.

You'll go deaf.

You'll go blind.

You'll become sterile or lose your sexual steam. ("A friend of mine told me that you could only ejaculate a hundred times in your life. I figured I only had about ten left when he told me. I was a little frightened that I had to spread them out over the next sixty years.")

It's a wonder—considering the enormous numbers of boys and girls, men and women who do masturbate —that the human race has continued to survive and procreate, and that we're not all deaf, blind, hairy-handed, toothless, pimple-faced, crippled, mindless, thumbless, hopeless, and beyond repair.

Virtually all these myths have been circulating for generations. So it's a wonder too that anyone continues to masturbate. But virtually everyone does, say the experts . . . starting around puberty, if not before.

Dr. Schreiner-Engel says: "Most women report that they started masturbating somewhere around puberty. And we know that about sixty-five percent of all adult women masturbate with some degree of frequency, and that almost all men masturbate." Pioneer sex researcher Alfred Kinsey "has the wonderful line," she says, "that ninety-nine percent of all men masturbate and one percent lie about it."

Among little kids, probably a hundred percent have touched themselves at least casually in an erotic and pleasurable way—which makes it a thoroughly normal behavior then, as well as in adolescence and in later years. Boys are more apt to "confess" to it than girls, who are much shyer about talking about it, perhaps because of the equally persistent myth that "girls don't masturbate."

Sex educators and therapists uniformly agree that masturbation is nothing for a parent to worry about; in fact it's downright good for the child. Still, the issue of masturbation is one that causes a lot of concern among parents, who, after all, grew up with all those myths. "I think that what parents worry about is based on the idea that you can masturbate too much and hurt yourself," reflects Dr. Cassell. "That's only fear. The body will take care of itself. Masturbation is not harmful at all."

The only thing harmful about masturbation is if you *think* it's harmful. In a word, guilt. All the fears kids pick up about masturbation don't necessarily deter them. These fears only serve to make the kids feel wretched about what they just did and will do again, no matter what they vow, because sex is an insistent drive. Like adults, children masturbate because it feels good and because it's comforting. But if they believe that what they are doing is definitely not okay, they end up suffering for their pleasure, which can have a sad influence on their developing sexuality. "The only possible danger of masturbation is the guilt associated with it," Dr. Lief reiterates.

Adolescents spend a lot of time worrying, "Am I normal?" and parents can step in and reassure them that if they masturbate they *are* normal. Parents can also contradict those enduring myths by telling the young ones, "No matter what Laura or Toby or Michael told you, you won't go nuts or turn gay or maim your penis or vagina or go blind."

To Mary Lee Tatum, "the most damaging myth about masturbation is that if you do masturbate regularly and enjoy it, it means that you can never have a good sexual relationship with another adult. That's terrible, awful...."

There's another myth, a brand-new one, that's gaining ground among some kids—kind of a Myth of the Eighties—and that is "If you *don't* masturbate you're not normal." Though most kids masturbate, not all of them do—and they should be told that's okay too.

What Percentage of Adolescents Masturbate?

Most of them do—and who's counting? By adulthood, about two-thirds of all women and virtually all men masturbate at least sometimes, say the statisticians. Conclusion: masturbation is here to stay. But the guilt that is frequently associated with it could turn out to be a real bummer. So include masturbation-is-okay in your sex chat, since your kids are probably wondering.

Can Any of These Forms of Sex Play Be Harmful to Your Child?

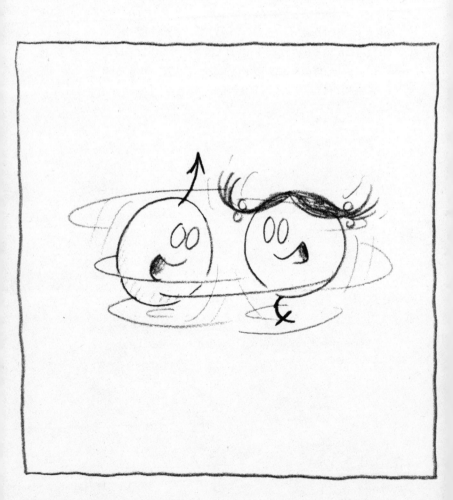

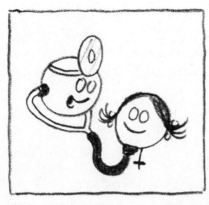

A. Playing doctor

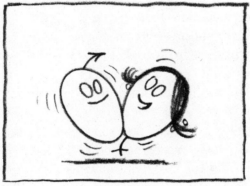

B. Pretend inter- course

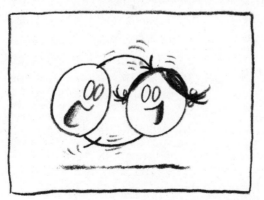

C. Mutual mastur- bation

D. None of the above

Imagine this. It's time for your little boy's afternoon treat. You knock on his door. "Timmy, dear," you say, "you've been in there a long time. You're missing your cookies and milk. What's going on in there, sweet pea?"

No answer.

"Um, Timmy, my sweet, why don't you answer?"

No answer. A burst of giggling.

"Timmy!"

"I'm playing with Barbie."

"Oh, well, then," you say reassured. Opening the door, you find that this is exactly what he is doing with his little next door neighbor—playing with her.

Shocked, horrified, and overwhelmed, you return to the kitchen. You proceed to eat all the kids' cookies, then an entire peach pie.

Question: Under the circumstances, do you feel that you are coping appropriately?

It's not easy being a parent, and some experiences seem to drive that home more than others. Okay, so masturbation's normal for kids—but how are you supposed to deal with it when they're behaving sexually with other kids, even kids of the same sex? Mutual masturbation, "pretend" intercourse, playing doctor— activities which kids engage in not only when they're little, but well into adolescence—are tough issues for parents, whose own parents probably didn't think too highly of these behaviors.

What that generation didn't know is that looking at, touching, and experimenting with each other's bodies is a normal part of growing up. "All kids play doctor in some form or another," says Dr. Carol Cassell. They play it with kids of the opposite sex, and they play it with kids of the same sex—not because they're "feeling sexy," but because they're just plain curious.

Playing, experimenting, mimicking, exploring—in these ways kids learn about the world, about themselves, and about each other. If they're just playing house instead of doctor and the little girl is dressing up in mommy's high heels and wants the little boy to wear her daddy's tie, we don't take them very seriously. But if the little girl wants them both to take off those clothes and make a baby, we call out the army. We forget they're just kids. "Sex play is very disturbing to parents," Mary Lee Tatum explains, "because we attribute adult motivation to child curiosity."

It isn't sex, it's playful curiosity.

Dr. Schreiner-Engel traces the way sex play among children normally develops. "First kids are enormously curious about their own bodies. Then around the age of seven or eight they become very curious about their friends' bodies, particularly the opposite sex, since somewhere along the line they've discovered that everybody does not look alike. You'll find that kids will work out opportunities to look at each other's bodies. Soon enough someone in the child's group of friends will have discovered that it feels good to touch someone's body. He or she tells all the friends and pretty soon everybody is experimenting. "

Sex play is, plain and simply, a learning opportunity for kids and a predictable part of their sexual development, although it may not be such a plain and simple issue for the parents to deal with. For some parents, the natural inclination is to break it up. Experts caution, however, that how you react to your kids' sex play with other kids is crucial, just as it is if you find them playing with their own bodies. Try not to overreact, in case you leave the child feeling guilty.

"These kids don't usually have any overriding sense

that their bodies are bad, or that they shouldn't be touched, or that no one's supposed to know that they do this," Dr. Schreiner-Engel explains. And why should they? "They're just enjoying their bodies, as it was meant to be."

If they are being inappropriately public about it, you might want to clue them in on some issues of privacy. But do try to keep your lid on, so they don't end up thinking they've just done something that will mark them for the rest of their lives.

The same is true when you catch two kids of the same sex playing with each other—a particularly tough one for parents to know how to deal with. Many parents jump to the conclusion that this means their child is homosexual—a natural assumption, perhaps, but a false one.

"Having homosexual contacts does not make one a homosexual," Dr. Gilmore says, a statement with which sex educators and therapists agree. "It is pretty normal for boys and boys and girls and girls to explore and to touch their own bodies." It is normal if your child is four, and it's just as normal if he or she is fourteen. Sex researcher Kinsey found, reports Dr. Harold Lief, that fully thirty-seven percent of all adolescent males, and somewhat fewer females, had had a sexual experience with someone of the same sex all the way to orgasm.

What do these statistics mean? "That parents should not be so upset by this kind of behavior," Dr. Lief says. "Obviously, thirty-seven percent of our male population isn't gay. The figure is actually somewhere between six and ten percent. So that means that at least two-thirds of those kids who had an orgastic experience with another boy have turned out to be hetero-sexual."

In other words, a child's sex experimentation at an early or late age has *no bearing* on his or her sexual orientation. And guilt and shame are more likely to do a child harm than any of the varieties of sex play kids come up with. You might pass that piece of infor-mation on to your kids. It will reassure them. Usually they don't think of their same-sex play as homosexual. But the kiddie sex grapevine being what it is, some children end up very worried that because they want to touch a friend of the same sex, or already have, that means they're gay. It doesn't. And it's normal—all the varieties of sex play among kids are normal.

. . . And all varieties of anxiety among parents, in-cluding overeating in times of stress, are also normal. But a plateful of chocolate-chip cookies and an entire peach pie is a bit much. Next time, our experts advise, skip the pie.

Can Any of These Forms of Sex Play Be Harmful to Your Child?

A. Playing doctor
B. Pretend intercourse
C. Mutual masturbation
*D. None of the above

While there's plenty of concern that children's sex play may be harmful, it's not. It's just a normal part of growing up.

When Do Kids Start Getting Interested in Sex?

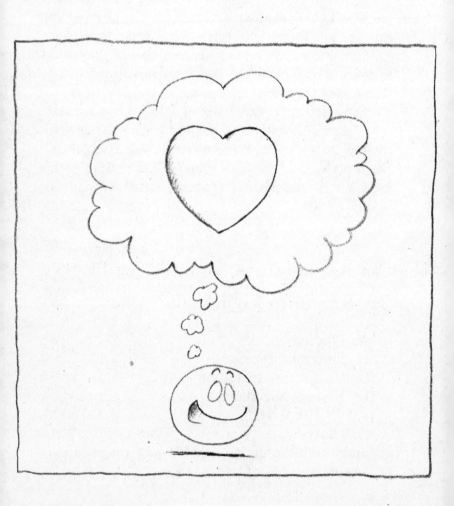

A. Three months

B. Three years

C. Eight to nine years

D. Twelve to thirteen years

It seems as if it happens overnight. One day he thinks girls are about as interesting as Brussels sprouts, and the next day his world is coming to an end because Joanie's line is still busy. "Why don't you talk to her in school tomorrow?" you ask, trying to co-opt the telephone for your own purposes. For this innocent question he casts you a dark look, and dials again. Still busy. He storms up to his room, turns on the radio, turns up the sound, turns it up even louder, and when you finally go to ask him to turn it down, you see him gyrating in front of the mirror, his shirt unbuttoned to his navel, combing and recombing his hair. Tomorrow, no doubt, you'll discover some "adult" magazines in the universal children's hiding place, under the mattress. And some condoms in his wallet.

Clearly his mind is no longer on his Legos. Or his homework.

"Would you turn that thing off and get to your homework?"

"Finished it!" he gloats, and snakes past you into his father's bathroom, to return reeking of expensive aftershave.

The phone rings. With a flying leap he takes off down the stairs. You don't race him. The phone hasn't been for you since s-e-x besieged your firstborn's brain cells. "Oh hi, Joanie!"

Judging from the downright hormonal behavior of adolescents, it does seem that interest in sex really begins for kids at puberty. But, say the experts, sex has been (and will continue to be) a central concern their whole lives. Even when they don't seem to care, kids are always aware of sex, and have had sexual thoughts and feelings, even sexual responses, from their earliest days.

Dr. Schreiner-Engel explains: "All infants are born with the capacity to become aroused. Males can have erections, females can lubricate, and all infants are born with the capacity to have orgasms. Many infants have orgasms while they're nursing or while they're pleasuring themselves. These innate capacities continue all the way through life until death—to become aroused, to have orgasm, and to have satisfaction or pleasure from sexual response. And that understanding, that the body is capable of sexual response," she says, "begins in infancy."

Dr. Shirley Zussman agrees: "There is a kind of interest and curiosity and readiness for sexual experience that occurs right from the very beginning." What kids understand and think about sex, though, and what they do about it, proceeds through various stages as they develop into young adults. And all the way along it's influenced by the messages they get from their parents and from society about what's "right" and "wrong" and about what it means to be sexual.

The more parents understand about their kids' awareness of sex and of the normal stages they need to pass through, the more they can help smooth the way into a healthy adult sexuality, say the experts. Each step of the way can have new anxieties for kids, especially if they have been getting conflicting or confusing messages from parents or from society.

Kids' earliest interest in sex is in the feelings they get from their own bodies. Their acceptance of their own bodies forms the foundation of their sexuality and sexual response throughout life. Soon comes their awareness of gender. By the time they are three, they know for sure that they are boys or girls. (If you want to test this out, Dr. Gilmore suggests you try telling a three-year-old girl what a nice boy she is and rate the indignance of her response.) Now comes a burning interest in the differences between their own bodies and other bodies. They want to touch their own bodies, and they want to know how other people, principally other kids, feel to the touch, too. They giggle and it's fun. While they do have sexual feelings in response to being touched, "they are not the same kinds of erotic feelings that you have as an adult," assures Dr. Cassell. Even when kids start getting boy crazy or girl crazy, or develop powerful and often agonizing crushes on adults of the opposite sex, all of which can happen at seven or eight or nine, they're not really attracted in the adult sense of the word. Eroticism, and complete adult sexual response and experience, has to wait for those hormones to begin to act in puberty.

While it used to be thought that kids went through a "latency phase" before puberty in which they weren't the least bit interested in or even aware of sex, sex experts now know beyond a doubt that kids never lose that interest. They may keep their feelings secret from their parents, though. Parents who don't think their kids are aware of their own sexuality aren't likely to bring the subject up for discussion. And in this atmosphere kids aren't likely to bring it up themselves —although by the time they are eight or nine they've been inundated with sexual information from the media or in the playground or on the streets. Better for the parents to explain, say sex therapists and educators, than for them to seek answers from their peers.

"You never know what the child is going to pick up," says Dr. Zussman, remembering a dinner party she went to some years ago at which the host's youngest son, who was about nine, trotted to the table in the middle of dinner to ask his father, "What does this mean?" "This" was a series of photographs of "fruits of the month" from a pornographic magazine, all depicting oral sex.

"The child had picked this up from his older brother's room. He had no awareness of what it was. His interest wasn't 'erotic'; he just wanted to know what these strange pictures meant. In the presence of a whole roomful of people, the father just picked up his son and put him on his lap and quietly explained to him. He didn't react with horror, he didn't tell the child to go away. He answered his son's question. It was done with such quiet calm that none of the rest of us knew what was being discussed until the father later told us. I've admired the man immensely ever since."

There's another aspect of sexuality that parents may not realize is on kids' minds, and that's their sexual roles. Even before kids are fully aware that they're boys or girls, they are getting the message from parents of how a little boy should act and how a little girl should act. "Many studies have been done that indicate that from absolute birth, as the neonate emerges from the womb, mommies treat boys and girls differently," reports Dr. Gilmore. The messages that parents and society wittingly or unwittingly give kids about what it means to be a girl and what it means to be a boy have terrific impact on how they end up thinking about themselves, how they act in relationships in adolescence and later in life, and how they feel about their bodies and their sexual response.

Sexual roles and sexual feelings all seem to explode upon kids (and their families!) at adolescence, as their hormones take over. Sex is at the forefront of their minds, even in their dreams. Now their sexual awareness is hard to miss. They way they dress, the way they act, the way they lust after one another, all point toward sexual interest in the way most adults are used to understanding it. Their sexual feelings take on an erotic component, and the chemistry of sexual attraction—the sex drive—at last begins.

But don't think that now that they are "mature" they don't need you anymore. More than ever, they need their parents (although they may not let you know that) to help make sense of these very bewildering changes in their bodies, their feelings, and their behavior. They're remarkably vulnerable. They're feeling a powerful sex drive, at the same time wondering, in Mary Lee Tatum's words, "What do I *do* with this?"

"A vast majority of our young people don't have any information about what they are going through," Dr. Gilmore mentions. "We know that very few parents, schools, or churches provide adequate sex information. Therefore, the kids are operating on a lot of myths out of television and *Playboy* and hearsay from the schoolyard. They don't really know what it is that they don't know. But, particularly if they are boys, from the time they are about ten, they have to pretend they know everything. Both boys and girls know they're supposed to be acting in a certain way, even though they are not quite sure what that way is, or why. Furthermore, they can't ask anybody."

Most of them think it's not a great subject to bring up at home. "And if they talk to each other, they have to lie to mask their own ignorance," Dr. Gilmore says, "because they think if they show their ignorance they'll be ridiculed. It's a really touchy time for kids."

Their bodies are probably giving them a hard time, too. When their bodies begin the slow process of change, the kids can become excruciatingly self-conscious. They think everybody's looking at them, or at the particular part of the body that they themselves are focused on, counting each pimple, judging each "flaw." "I think a parent has to understand," explains Dr. Gilmore, "that while a child may seem calm on the outside, there may be a lot of distress and a lot of concern inside."

Although kids' interest in sex becomes most apparent when they enter their teens, it's been there since infancy. What they think and how they act about it will change as they go through all the phases and stages of childhood. It's a continuing process of development, and easier for kids when parents can encourage them to understand and feel okay about that interest. Concern about sex isn't unique to adolescents. Preteens, little kids, babies—we're all coping with sexual experience from the very beginning of our existences. "Sexuality is something that emerges over the whole life cycle," states Dr. Zussman. Thus, adults might be expected to have one or two concerns on the subject themselves!

When Do Kids Start Getting Interested in Sex?

*A. **Three months**
 B. Three years
 C. Eight to nine years
 D. Twelve to thirteen years

When Do Girls Become Sexually Mature and Old Enough to Conceive?

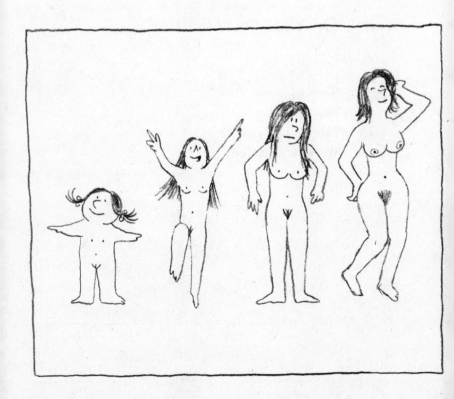

A. Nine

B. Twelve

C. Fourteen

D. Sixteen

Having the curse, falling off a log, getting your dog, your aunt Mary's come to tea—these are but four of the expressions adolescent girls have used over the years to communicate to one another that they have their periods.

"In gym class we used to call it 'monthly,'" recalls a forty-year-old Missouri mother of three. "This would excuse us from the mandatory showers. I hated those showers. Even if I used a shower cap, they'd destroy the hairdo that I had painfully preserved through a long sleepless night bound up in rollers with brushes in them, and clips and bobby pins and hairnets. So I'd have my 'monthly' fairly frequently. Then they started keeping records. One day the gym teacher asked me to stay after class. She suggested with a sugary sweet voice that she was terribly concerned for my health and thought that we should phone my mother and tell her that I seemed to be menstruating (only gym and hygiene teachers ever used *that* word) every fourteen days for ten days at a time. Of course I couldn't have her do that. For one thing, my mother knew that I hadn't even gotten my period. . . ."

She finally did begin to menstruate when she was fourteen. By that time she believed herself fairly sophisticated about such matters, as her best friend had been regularly falling off a log since she was eleven and a half. "She had real honest-to-goodness breasts in seventh grade. Some of the boys used to snigger about how 'developed' she was. But she carried it off pretty well. By eighth grade I was really jealous. So one day I asked her if I could borrow her bra—she wore a 34C. I stuffed it with Kleenex and put it on under my sweater. I sauntered down to breakfast thinking that my parents would simply conclude that I'd grown. My mother was pretty cool, but my father did a big double take and demanded that I go and take off those 'falsies.' Falsies! I was really hurt that he thought they weren't mine."

No two girls, then as now, have the same pattern of growth or experience during adolescence. Looking back, it's easy to laugh about it all, but while you're going through it, these differences can be mortifying. On average, menarche (the first menstrual period) occurs when a girl is twelve and a half years old. But the range of ages that this average represents swings from as early as eight to late in the teens, all of which is considered normal, although the kids themselves may not think so. The very young child who has not yet been taught about menstruation may believe she's bleeding to death, and the sixteen-year-old who has yet to get her period may fear she's backward and under-developed for life.

Adolescents can suffer devastating anxiety when they think, as so many boys and girls do during these years, that there is something "wrong" with them. They think that they are developing too fast, too slowly, or incorrectly. In Dr. Lief's experience, "It's almost universal for males to have some anxiety about penis size and for girls to worry about how their breasts are developing, not only in size and shape but in sym-metry."

"A lot of the anxieties kids go through at this time needn't be," insists Mary Lee Tatum. The anxiety can be avoided if kids have the right kind of information about this time of their lives, about how each person develops differently, and about what the process in-cludes and how long it takes to complete. "One has to allow time for this maturation to occur," states Dr. Lief. "With girls, you have to wait until at least fifteen to see whether there's any truly significant problem with the development of breasts"—which there usually isn't.

Educator Tatum believes that parents could help their kids significantly if they would "point out all the differences and stress how wonderful it is that human beings have so many of them."

Puberty neither begins nor ends suddenly. Over three to four years, a girl's body changes in both subtle and obvious ways. Her breasts begin to grow, her genitals to thicken; she develops "axillary hair" under her arms and on her legs, and pubic hair. Her body begins to take on a new shape, and eventually the first egg is released from her ovaries, resulting in her first menstrual period and signaling her capacity to conceive a child (though not necessarily to bear a healthy child to term or to adequately care for it once it is born).

"Menstruation is an exceedingly important time in a girl's life," says Dr. Schreiner-Engel. "It is a major transition point in this whole puberty phase. I think it ought to be celebrated." And celebrate she did, each time one of her own three daughters reached puberty. "When my oldest daughter reached menstruation and came to tell me about it, I hugged her and congratulated her and then told her to pick a restaurant, because the whole family was going to go out and celebrate.

"She was really surprised and delighted. She picked her favorite restaurant. The whole family—all five kids, grandparents—went out and toasted her. And her reaction was, 'Wow! This is really neat. It's really good to grow up.'"

The physical changes that precede puberty continue after the onset of menstruation, as do the corresponding and often bewildering (to both parents and daughters) psychological and emotional changes. A girl is much more aware now of being female, of her body, of her attractiveness. And she becomes oh so aware of the boys out there and of their being *male*. Her sex drive is keenly felt, her thoughts turn to romance . . . and her parents' thoughts frequently turn to terror. Sexual maturity means sex, doesn't it? How far is she going to go? With whom? Can they interfere? Can they even offer advice? And if they do, will she listen?

If sex has been an open topic in the household, by all means keep on talking. And if it hasn't, better to open it up for discussion right now. "This is a time when a child becomes sexually mature and can become a parent," stresses Dr. Gilmore. "It is crucial for every child to understand how reproduction takes place and that if she has sexual intercourse, there is a likelihood that a child will result from that."

Information, information, information, the experts urge—truthful information, of course, offered with your honest feelings and willingness to engage in discussion. Try to avoid scare tactics. Attempting to terrorize your daughter out of engaging in sexual activity, while admittedly a tempting thought for a parent from time to time, isn't likely to stop her. Either she'll end up feeling guilty about what she does anyway or she'll do it to defy you.

"I did that—defied my mother," says our friend in Missouri. "She thought that my boyfriend and I were staying out too late, and she tried to scare me into thinking that I'd 'get a reputation.' I was sixteen and I managed to sneak out one night after my parents were asleep. My boyfriend was waiting in his car and we drove around for a while then parked and made out. He asked whether I thought we should go all the way. I said I didn't think so. And he asked, well then what were we going to do for the rest of the night. I couldn't think of anything, so I went back home. Word got out in school about our big night out and about my virtuous behavior. I was terribly embarrassed. I didn't mind being a virgin, but I didn't want to seem excessive about it. So I guess the moral of the story is: Watch out, girls, or you may prove your mothers right. It took me years to get rid of the reputation I earned that night!"

When Do Girls Become Sexually Mature and Old Enough to Conceive?

A. Nine
*B. Twelve
C. Fourteen
D. Sixteen

The average age for girls to start menstruating is somewhere around twelve years old. But the range is very wide—anywhere from eight to eighteen—and the actual process of physical and emotional maturation takes a long time. Your daughter needs love, encouragement, support—and plenty of real and realistic information.

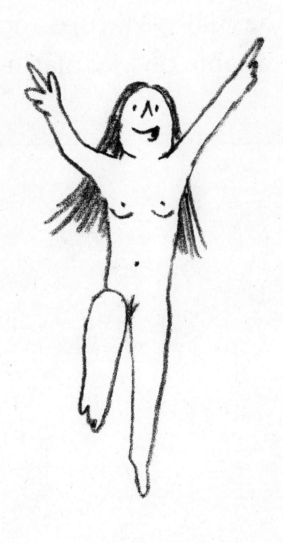

When Are Boys Sexually Mature and Capable of Ejaculating?

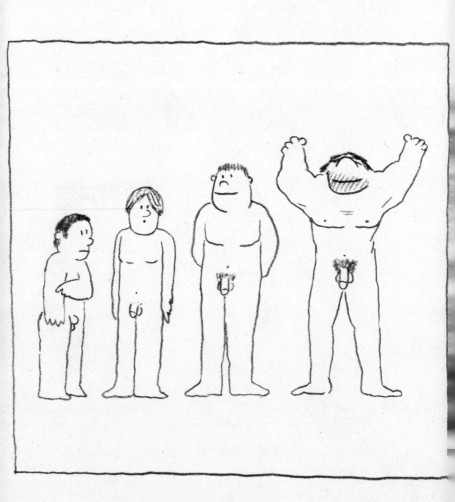

A. Nine

B. Eleven

C. Thirteen

D. Fifteen

Boys have the reputation of being late bloomers, sexual and social laggards, mere babies compared to their pubescent female counterparts.

Jim's now thirty-four, but when he was a teenager he thought he must be sexually retarded, it took him so long to mature:

"When I was fifteen I was the only kid in my group of best buddies who hadn't matured yet. My voice was just beginning to crack, I felt like I was covered with baby fat, but that wasn't the worst of it. The other three boys started staging tournaments in the woods behind school to see who could ejaculate the farthest. At least they said they did. Humiliation of humiliations, I couldn't even compete. And if they weren't doing that, they were hanging around with girls. Well,

I wasn't much good in the girls department either. They could have cared less about me. So I'd just mope along home in despair. No wet dreams, even."

Jim had a new French teacher that year. She had recently come to the United States from Paris. Jim began to notice that she was very sexy, which wasn't the kind of thought he was used to having, and that she wore intoxicating, delicate, sweet perfume. In no time, he was madly in love with her. Now, every day after school the lovestruck youth, whose voice was fast deepening, would race home from school to be "alone" with Mademoiselle in his room. When his mother would ask what on earth he was doing in there, Jim would respond with an indignant, often breathless, "Nothing!"

Mademoiselle had noticed Jim, too. One day she asked him to stay after class, to tell him how much she thought his performance in class had improved. Walking him to the door, she put her arm around him and gave him a little squeeze. Jim inhaled her perfume so deeply, his knees went weak. After school, he could hardly make it home to his room.

The next morning Jim awoke with the best feeling of his whole life. He knew he had had a dream about Mademoiselle, although he couldn't remember the details. Suddenly he realized something felt kind of funny, wet and sticky. Could it be . . . ? He needed to make sure. With his mother at the door insisting if he didn't get up he'd be late for school, Jim discovered for sure: "What a man!"

Jim didn't join his friends in their boyish contests. "After Mademoiselle I figured I was too mature for that," he said, laughing. And he didn't return to afternoons in his room. "You see, there was this girl who sat near me in French. She asked me if I could help her with her homework. She wore perfume, too. So we started going to her house after school, and now it was her mom who wanted to know what was going on in there. 'French vocabulary!' she'd gasp. That was true," Jim says wistfully. *La femme*, woman. *L'homme*, man. *Baiser*, to kiss. *Aimer*, to love. . . ."

Jim was nearly sixteen when he reached sexual maturity, and he certainly made up for lost time But he hadn't been the "sexual retard" that he feared he was. In our culture the average age for boys to reach sexual maturity is thirteen and a half, but the range of what is considered normal is as wide as it is for girls.

"There ought to be a big T-shirt for kids to wear that says in neon letters: AM I NORMAL? Because kids worry incredibly about that," says Dr. Cassell, adding, "We have this myth that somewhere there is truly a norm—that when you're thirteen you're absolutely going to look a certain way and feel a certain way and be something different from the way you were at twelve. Kids worry, 'When is this normal thing going to happen to me? Am I normal?' "

The truth is, in adolescence *everything* is normal. No two kids have identical experiences.

"I think the best that parents can do," Dr. Cassell concludes, "is to let each kid know that he or she is perfectly normal for *him* or *her*." Different people just develop at different rates. "You're developing at your own speed, you'll get there, and I love you whether you have big square muscles or baby fat" is the reassuring message kids need to hear early on from their parents.

For boys and girls, adolescence is a time when they need to feel most like everybody else, although in reality it's a time when they're most different. One fifteen-year-old may be panting after girls and they're panting after him, while his best friend doesn't understand those feelings at all, yet feels rejected because he isn't receiving the same attention.

Don't wait for your half-man/half-boy to ask what in the world is going on with him. At this age, many boys have to act as if they know everything there is to know about sex and sexuality and are petrified that the true extent of their ignorance will be uncovered. That doesn't mean you can't hand them a good book.

As in girls, the changes in boys that signal puberty occur over a period of years, before and after the time they become capable of ejaculating (in other words, capable of impregnating a female). Their testicles descend, their scrotum and penis grow larger, they develop hair on their body including the pubic region and face. Their voices begin to deepen, their muscle structures to change, their height to increase. Some time before they're out of their teens, the process is complete, but when each step will happen is impossible to predict. And a lot of things can happen that seem pretty weird.

Dr. Harold Lief tells what happened to him early in his teens:

"I had an experience that I'm sure is paralleled by thousands of boys. I can remember when I was past twelve I had some slight increase in the size of my breasts, which were also tender. I know now that this condition is called 'temporary gynecomastia,' which is the technical term for the swelling of the breasts, and that it's perfectly normal; at least fifty percent of boys have this experience.

"But I remember thinking, 'My God! I'm turning into a female!' I was embarrassed to go out. I was afraid that my peers would see these little breast buds and ridicule me."

Eventually the swelling stopped and his adolescent body returned to normal. But the experience took its toll. "I'm sure," he says, "that so many adolescents can be helped with this if they are informed that these are normal experiences and nothing to be ashamed of."

And it's perfectly normal for boys to mature, sexually and socially, later than girls. There is a year's difference in the average ages at which they reach sexual maturity, "and this creates a tremendous gap between boys and girls between seventh and ninth grade," Mary Lee Tatum points out. "The girls will be going around saying, 'Oh, they're so *immature*,' and the boys will be trying as best they can to look down on the girls, saying, 'They're so out of it.' "

But the truth is, many of them are immature in comparison, which must be taken into account by teachers and parents too. In adolescence, boys need just as much information—about reproduction, bodies, feelings, sexually transmitted diseases, responsibility —as girls do. However, says Dr. Lief, because of the immaturity factor, boys may not be able to absorb it as readily as girls do. So keep plugging.

Maturity means so much more than sexual capability. There's emotional maturity, social maturity, intellectual maturity. Boys and girls go at their own pace, and each individual has a unique pace besides. Eventually they all grow up. Then you'll be saying, "How time flies!"

When Are Boys Sexually Mature and Capable of Ejaculating?

    A. Nine
    B. Eleven
*C. **Thirteen**
    D. Fifteen

Adolescence is a difficult time. The experts tell us that boys reach puberty at the average age of thirteen and a half, but as with girls, the maturing process isn't complete just yet.

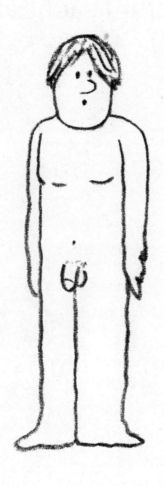

Does It Matter Which Parent Teaches the Kids About Sex?

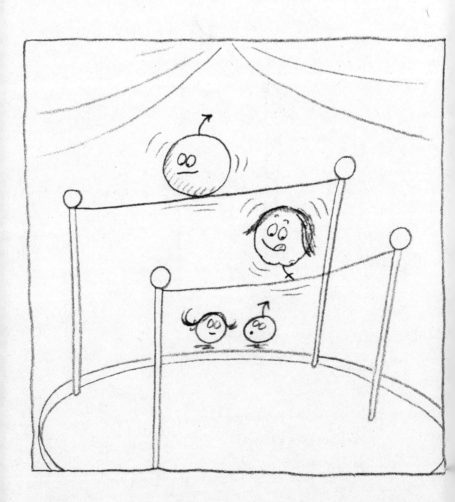

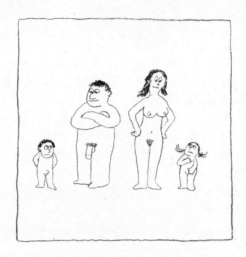

A. Girls need to hear from their moms, and boys from their dads

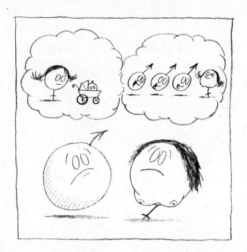

B. Boys can learn from their mothers, and girls from their fathers

C. It doesn't matter who teaches what to whom, as long as somebody does it

D. All of the above

"Daddy, what's a clitoris?"

"Is that you Sandra, or is it Davey? I can't hear with the water running."

"It's Sandy."

Gerald opens the bathroom door and lets his daughter in. "What's that you wanted to know, honey?"

"What's a clitoris?"

"Well, darling, I think that's a question you should ask your mother."

Gerald returns to his shaving. A few minutes pass.

"Daddy, what's a clitoris?"

"That you, Davey?"

"Yeah. Sandy said she's got this thing inside her that makes her feel good. She says it's just like my penis only it's better, because she can't pee in her pants with it. Is that true, Daddy? Does Sandy have a better penis than I do?"

"What did your mother say?"

"She said I should ask you," said the boy, breaking into sobs.

"Now, now, don't cry, Davey. Sandy doesn't have a penis. Only you do. And look how big it is. I bet you've never seen something like that on your sister, now, have you?"

"No." David's sobs cease. "Then what's a clitoris?"

"It's just this little thing. Ask your mother."

"I *told* you already—she said to ask *you*."

"Tell her my contract says I only have to do penises," says Gerald. "No clitorises, no windows, and no fancy cooking."

Traditionally, in our culture, it's been the mother who has introduced the subject of sex and answered the kids' questions, especially in the early years. Dr. Gilmore says: "All the studies that I know of about sex education in the home indicate that the mothers are by far the greater conveyors of information about sexuality. Fathers almost never do it."

The way the baby is held, fed, bathed, fondled, and comforted establishes the fundamental trust a child will have in his or her own body and in contact with other people. In turn, this trust forms the basis of all future sexuality. In our culture, holding and handling the baby is most often the mother's responsibility. This puts her "in charge" of the most important aspects of sexual learning that the child will receive in his or her life—much more important, Dr. Lief believes, than anything that is ever said about sex later.

Teaching control of bodily functions, toilet training, feeding, usually are mothers' jobs, too, and attitudes toward kids' enjoyment in making a mess, says Dr. Lief, "have a profound effect on the way they end up looking at their bodies and their appetites."

But it doesn't have to be mom who alone bears these enormous responsibilities. "Variation in this pattern would be great," he says. "The child has two parents. So much the better if both feel free and easy about bodily contact and bodily functions."

Sexual learning takes place in many ways. The experts are in strong agreement that fathers and mothers have distinct and different contributions to make to their kids' understanding of sex and to their developing sexuality. "Both genders need both genders," Dr. Carol Cassell asserts. "You get messages about your sexuality—being masculine or feminine—from the parent of the opposite sex. And you get your role model of how to be a woman or a man from the parent of the same sex. So it's very important that each parent realizes that he or she indeed has a different part to play. Maleness is different from femaleness—and that has nothing to do with superiority, simply biological differences. Each parent brings a richness to that perspective."

Mary Lee Tatum adds: "Opposite-sex and same-sex approval are both very important. Everybody wants to know, 'Am I attractive?' 'Is being a woman a good thing?' 'Is being a man a good thing?' 'What does it mean to be a woman or a man?'" All these questions are answered by both parents in one way or another.

As puberty approaches, for example, a girl needs her mom. That's not only because mom can clarify physiology and hygiene, some of which the child may already have learned in school. Mostly a girl needs her mother because her mother "has experienced the maturing process and can share her feelings about it and what it means, and answer questions more specifically about bodily feelings," says Dr. Shirley Zussman.

But she needs her dad too. She needs his acknowledgment of this so-important time of her life. Mary Lee Tatum believes "it would be wonderful if a father could bring home a bouquet of roses for his daughter when she began to menstruate."

"The father is the girl's first boyfriend," says Dr. Schreiner-Engel. "The way he reacts to her, the way he treats her, is what she learns to expect from men the rest of her life. If her father expresses appreciation of her, expresses pride, shows that he cares for her, that he sees her as a wonderful little girl and a beautiful developing woman, a capable woman—these are attitudes that she's going to take about herself and expect of men in relationships from then on."

Equally, a boy needs both his father's and mother's

support during this crucial time. Unfortunately, boys are frequently left out by both parents. "There's this kind of backslapping male camaraderie that assumes boys sort of pick this stuff up," says Dr. Gilmore. Usually girls are prepared to some extent for menstruation, but nobody tells boys about wet dreams and ejaculations, which may turn out to be a frightening surprise.

When it comes to providing explicit information to your kids about sex, most of the educators agree that there are no hard and fast rules about who should talk to whom about what. "Ideally," says Dr. Gilmore, in addition to man to man and woman to woman, "fathers should be able to talk to daughters, and mothers to sons, at least part of the time, so that a child has a chance to get information about sex from a person of the opposite sex who's safe."

But, he quickly adds, comfort is the deciding factor, for both the parent and the child. If one parent is really uncomfortable and can't get the words out, the parent who is more comfortable with it should do it, no matter the sex of the child. Kids are, after all, better at reading attitudes than at hearing words.

There's no reason why a father couldn't discuss menstruation, for example, with his daughter if he's comfortable, believes Dr. Lief. Even so, she may be embarrassed. "You have to look at the interaction," he says. Adolescence is a time of very delicate feelings between girls and their dads. A mutual comfort level may be very difficult to achieve. In that case it's better to leave the specific birds-and-bees material to mom, with dad making sure to support the child's newfound maturity.

One thing dads can talk to their daughters about,

though, is love, sex, and sexuality from the male point of view. "I think it's very important for the father to talk to his young son about being a man, and what his vision of that is. And it is just as important," insists Dr. Cassell, "to discuss with the young woman what men think and feel, what male sexuality is like."

The same goes for mothers and sons. Once the boy understands the mechanics of the sex act, how much fuller his understanding will be if he can hear what it feels like from the woman's point of view. Educators point out that the older the kids get, the more interested they are in exploring feelings, relationships, the deeper meanings of things.

Single-parent households need not be at a disadvantage, as long as there's a role model of the opposite sex who is involved with the kids. "Kids are amazingly resilient," says Mary Lee Tatum. "They generally find role models for themselves outside the family. That will usually happen in school, when teacher becomes God."

To provide some opposite-sex continuity for the whole family, the experts recommend supplying someone of the "missing" sex to provide the absent perspective. In families in which the father is no longer present, girls need the approval of an adult man who's important to them, and they need to learn how to be at ease with the opposite sex. Boys also need that all-important model and person to do "man things" with as well as somebody to turn to if they want for information about sex and their changing bodies.

"If a woman is raising a child alone, I think that she has to make a real effort to have male companions who are friendly in an extended family way with her and her children," says Dr. Cassell. These should not be men with whom she is interested in having a sexual relationship, whose presence in the kids' life is likely to be subject to the whims of romance. A Dutch uncle type with a long-term allegiance to your kids is best: "Just a nice guy who'll come over to the house and spend casual time. He doesn't have to go out in the backyard and play catch with your sons. He can just talk about what his day is like and what he's interested in, about who he is."

Does It Matter Which Parent Teaches the Kids About Sex?

A. Girls need to hear from their moms, and boys from their dads
B. Boys can learn from their mothers, and girls from their fathers
C. It doesn't matter who teaches what to whom, as long as somebody does it
*D. **All of the above**

Kids learn about sex and what it means to be a boy or a girl from both their parents. They need to talk to mom and to dad and to feel that both are with them all the way as they mature sexually. But the most important thing is that the parents should feel comfortable talking sex with their kids. It's okay too, say the experts, if the parent who's more comfortable does most of the talking.

Question 15

Should Parents Teach
Their Own Sexual
Values to Their Kids?

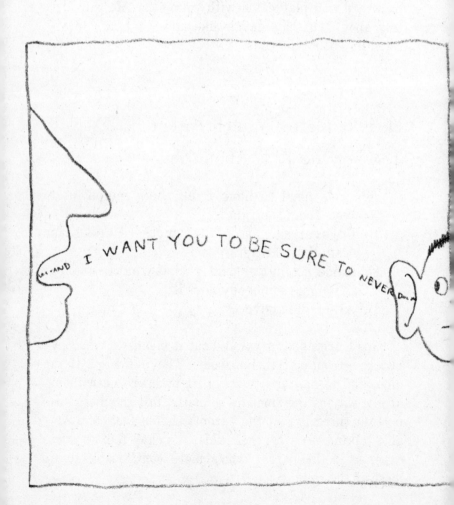

A. Yes

B. No

I am thy parent who brought thee out of the womb into the world of sexual responsibility and thou shalt respect what I have to say about that.

Thou shalt have no sex until thou art grown and fully capable of dealing with it and its consequences.

Thou shalt get none of thy ideas about sex from song lyrics.

Thou shalt ensure that thy sexual behavior never takes advantage of another human being.

Whosoever claimeth that sex and drugs are a worthwhile combination thou shalt cast out of the land.

Thou shalt not present thy parents with a grandchild until they are ready.

Thou shalt love thy partner as thyself, and thy partner's body as thy own.

Thou shalt respect the married state and seek it for thyself.

Whatsoever showeth that women were created to be pretty and men to be tough shall make thee think twice about that.

All these things being done, thou shalt find fulfillment in love, in work, in sex all the days of thy life.

Moses came down the mountain with the Ten Commandments and found everybody worshiping a golden calf. He found this very discouraging. In a temper he threw down the tablet and broke it. A lot of parents know this feeling. What's the use of laying down the moral law when the kiddies are worshiping their rock or "punk" idols?

"Parents are struggling to deal with a world of changing sexual values," states Dr. Cassell. What they think is right and wrong is often very, very different from what kids may pick up from their peers. Some parents conclude that since the kids' world is so "new," it's best to let them go their own way without any old-fashioned and sure-to-be-resented interference. Other parents choose a stricter course, attempting to impose their own sets of values on kids who will not heed them.

"You're damned if you do and damned if you don't," Dr. Gilmore concedes. "If you try to impose values, any kid with a reasonably healthy ego will do the opposite. And if you're completely permissive, the kids think you don't really love them and will go off and become promiscuous or get pregnant, just to demonstrate that they're important."

What's a parent to do?

Dr. Lief says, "Parents have an obligation to put

their values across, but in a nondemanding way: 'This is what I think. This is what I prefer. This is what I recommend. These are the pros and cons of my approach. These are the pros and cons of another approach.' "

But will the kids listen? Parents may not realize that information about what they value, what preferences and choices they make, how they go about making them, are all very useful to kids when they make their own decisions, says Dr. Lief. "And what we're after here is responsible decision making."

The key word, say the experts, is *nondemanding*. Sharing your sexual values and ethical positions "doesn't mean imposing them, but simply saying, 'I don't expect that this is necessarily how you're going to feel or think or act, but I would like you to know how I feel about it. This is where I come from in terms of my morality and my point of view.' It's not very different," says Dr. Zussman, "from the way you would express your other values about all aspects of living, about honesty, behaving responsibly for your actions in relation to other people, about education, about anything."

It's hard, she admits, not to insist on your own values and ways of looking at sexual conduct, because parents always want the best for their kids. When the young adolescent child wants to have intercourse, most parents will feel that this is certainly not in his or her best interests. Say precisely that, in no uncertain terms, she recommends, but remember that kids end up making their own decisions no matter what you do. If you express your own sincere point of view, you'll give the child a chance to ask questions and express his or her feelings and you can talk about it. But if you try to "force it down their throats," says Dr. Zussman, they'll just go off and rebel. This is the nature of normal, healthy adolescence.

"You *can* say, 'Look, I really don't *want* you to have sexual intercourse,' " Dr. Gilmore explains. "Be very specific about it. 'You're not old enough for it. You're not ready for it. The consequences are terrible, and here's what they are. . . .' It's a relief for a lot of kids to have their parents tell them that. It gets them off the hook." When they get in the back of the car and have to decide what's going to happen next, they can take the burden off themselves by saying or thinking, 'Mommy doesn't want me to do that.' "

Kids may not realize just how many points of view there really are about most of the important issues of life. In addition to what they themselves think, parents can help by pointing out the various and varying messages about sexual values and lifestyles that are delivered by religions, government, magazines, movies, TV, books, schools, rock song lyrics, famous people, and people whom they know. Kids will begin to see that the choices are not limited to "what my friends say and what my parents say." And discussing the pros and cons of each will give the family a whole lot to talk about.

Parents, too, may have more choices than they think. In addition to permissive and overcontrolled parenting styles, says Dr. Gilmore, there's a third style, which one researcher calls "authoritative" (*not* authoritarian!). Authoritative parents "make very clear what their values are about sexuality and other moral and ethical issues. Though they make their positions strongly known, they really do leave the choosing up to the child," says the educator.

Research shows that parents who adopt this style "tend to produce kids who are independent thinkers and moral and ethical thinkers, even though, of course, they do make mistakes. They will tend not to be promiscuous or uncontrolled, nor will they be overcontrolled and too rigorous in suppressing their own sexuality."

But there's a lot more to teaching sexual values than talking about them. The truth is, your kids are learning sexual values from you from their earliest awareness. How parents relate to each other, how they touch each other and the kids, how they react to their kids' developing sexuality, what they think about how boys and girls are supposed to behave, how they react to other people—all this and more forms the basis from which kids develop their own sexual values, emphasizes Mary Lee Tatum. Parents can teach sexual values "certainly by living what they want their child to adopt, which isn't always easy," she adds, "especially for single parents."

Remember that *not* talking about it also imparts a sexual value. To a child, silence translates to mean sex is not something people should be open about (and if you have any questions about sexual decisions, you can't ask anybody for help).

It's best to launch in early, recommend the educators and therapists, so that a lot of these issues—such as how you feel about birth control—can be discussed at the appropriate time without a whole lot of tension and anxiety. These discussions then become part of a continuing process instead of what comes out sounding like a stern moral lecture when the kids are in their teens.

Say what you have to say and stick by the kids and hope for the best. Remember, Moses was not a patient man, but *he* hung in there.

Should Parents Teach Their Own Sexual Values to Their Kids?

*A. Yes
  B. No

It couldn't be more important, the experts say. Even though the world of sexual values seems to have been turned on its head, kids need to know exactly what their parents feel is right in order to make responsible decisions on their own behalf. They'll respect you for it.

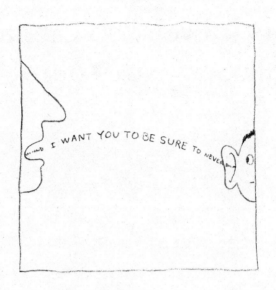

Is It Ever Too Late to Talk Sex with Your Kids?

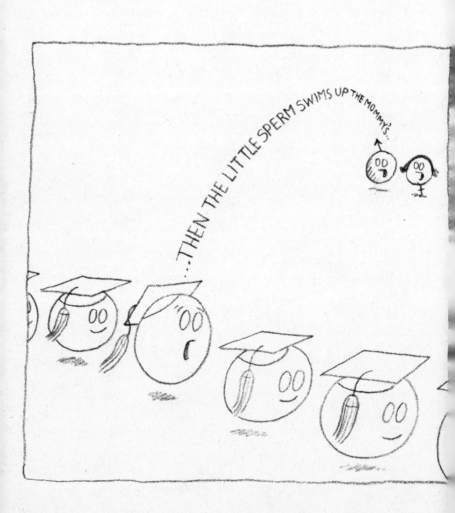

A. Yes

B. No

Talking sex with your kids—no one said it's easy. But the earlier you start the better. As time goes by, there's as much to unlearn as there is to learn. And what if you haven't really broached the subject? Is it ever too late to start?

"Howard, dear, this is your mother."

"Oh hi, Mom. What are you doing calling so late? It's almost midnight. We're in bed."

"I'm sorry, dear, but I just had to call. I know you and Arlene have been trying to have a baby for such a long time. Your father says it's my fault, that I didn't explain things right when you were a child. . . . Howard, what's all that noise? Is this a bad connection?"

"It's the birds and the bees," her son answered. "The phone started them up again."

"I'm interrupting?" Howard's mother asked shyly.

"That's okay," he told her. "This goes on every night. We let the birds out of their cage, and the bees out of the box we keep them in. Then we climb under the netting. We're really determined, Mom. It's just like you explained—"

"Oh dear, your father always said you'd take me literally."

Howard's mother began to explain things a little more realistically.

In the morning Howard was a new man. He got up and opened the window and let all the birds and bees out. Arlene couldn't imagine what he was doing. So he told her what his mother had told him. Arlene had never had much faith in the birds and the bees anyhow. Her mother had explained where kids came from differently.

"Does that mean . . . ?" she began.

But Howard had anticipated his wife's question. "Right," he said, drawing her in his arms, "cancel the stork order."

"It's never too late to talk about sex," says Dr. Lief, "even with a *ninety*-year-old. Everyone is interested in sex till his or her dying day. It's the subject about which we have more interest, generally speaking, than any other subject in life. It's never too late to talk to anybody about sex if it's done in a sensible, dignified fashion."

There are lots of very human reasons why many parents don't get around to talking sex with their kids. For one, they just don't know what to say. They feel inadequate. Kids today live in such a different world from the one parents grew up in. Sometimes it seems the language they speak isn't even the same.

Dr. Schreiner-Engel agrees that "most of us never had the kind of sex education that we're now trying to provide for our own children." But there's no reason, she says, "why the parent even has to know the answer or have all the right information." There are so many good books around aimed at each age group that parents and kids can go through them together. And parents can get some books for themselves, too.

It is much less important for parents to know the "right" answer than for them to convey that they're interested in talking about the whole subject, and that they're available to answer questions and help in solving problems.

But what if your kid is one of those who doesn't ask questions? That's another big reason why parents may never get around to the subject.

"It's really common for parents to say, 'I've been wanting to have a talk with my child but I've been waiting till I'm asked a question,'" says Dr. Cassell. "One time I asked a parent, 'Well, how old is your child?' and he said, 'My son is seventeen, and I don't think he's ever been interested because he's never asked me anything.'"

Kids may not ask questions for lots of reasons. Maybe they think *you* don't want to talk about it, or that the subject is off-limits, or they're embarrassed. The more silent you and they are about the subject, the more convinced they'll be that it's just not the right kind of thing to bring up. But they're interested, all right, exceedingly.

You may be embarrassed yourself, especially if your kids are older and sex has never been a free and easy subject in your house. Or you may be afraid you gave them all the wrong information years ago and you'll not be able to give them what they really need now. Parents worry so!

"You can't harm your kids showing them you are only human, can you?" queries Dr. Cassell. If you're embarrassed, say so. "The best thing that kids like to know is that parents are people. What stops parents is that they're so afraid of saying the wrong thing. And the right thing is just what you're thinking and what you're feeling. It's never too late to sit down and talk to your child, no matter how old he or she is, about your feelings about human sexuality."

Afraid you have already said the wrong thing— filled the child's head with notions about sex that you don't think are true anymore, or you wish you hadn't said? Mary Lee Tatum suggests: "Try saying, 'You know, honey, I don't feel so good about what I did or said about this issue five years ago. What do you think? Let's talk about it now.' There's nothing that builds self-esteem in an adolescent as much as being talked to as if he or she had adult capacity to think—which they do," she adds.

Being able to talk to your child about sex means being able to talk about relationships and self-esteem, pleasure, parenthood, human values, goals, responsibilities, warmth, love, giving, and about the birds and bees, figuratively speaking.

Is It Ever Too Late to Talk Sex with Your Kids?

A. Yes
*B. No

While it's true it's never too late to talk sex with your kids, it's also true it's never too early. Children are naturally curious. Answering their questions about sex won't always be easy, but kids really want to learn about the subject from their parents. And they don't just want to know about the mechanics. They want to know what it means. They are as interested in the feelings of love as they are in lovemaking. So answer their questions the best way you can. Help your kids make sense of the information bombarding them from all directions.

Today's a good day. Why wait?

How Do You Break the Ice in Talking Sex with Your Kids?

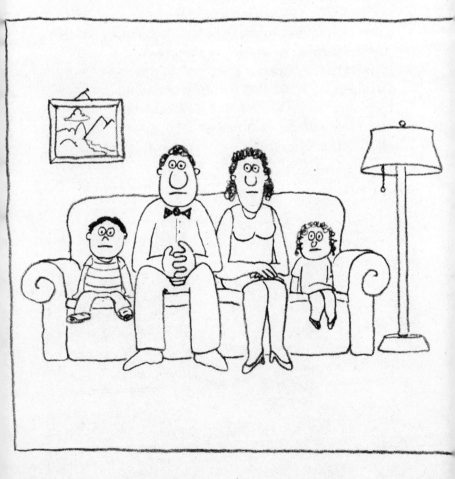

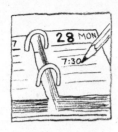 **A.** Schedule a talk

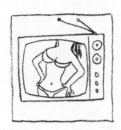 **B.** Turn on the TV

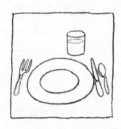 **C.** Bring it up at dinner

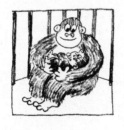 **D.** Go to the zoo

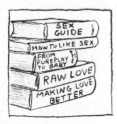 **E.** Give them books to read

F. All of the above

Consider option A:

MEMO TO: All children

FROM: Your parents

CONCERNING: Sex

MESSAGE: A conference is being held after break-
           fast on Saturday on the back porch to
           acquaint all members of this household
           who are between six and twelve years
           old with the facts of life. You will
           please appear promptly at 9:30 after
           you have cleaned your rooms. Atten-
           dance is mandatory. Crayons will be
           provided.

Too formal for your house, you say? Then try option B:

"Henry, honey, do you have the TV listings? I want
to know when that sex-education show for kids is on.
I'm sure I saw something about it in the paper. It's supposed to be very good."

"Unh, unh, haven't seen them. Anyway, I think that
show was on last week."

"Oh no—and here I was hoping I could just sit them
down in front of the television and they'd learn everything about sex without us having to talk about it. Now
what are we going to do, Henry?"

"Have 'em watch 'Dallas.' That should do it."

If that is not the kind of sex education you had in
mind, move directly to option C—the dinner table. One
dad we know figured he had enough courage for that
particular approach. He'd just come home from the
office, sit down, and kind of free-associate:

"This is a wonderful dinner, honey. The steak's done to a perfect medium rare—that's hard to do, kids, I don't know if you realize that. But when you grow up and start cooking, you'll find out that a steak goes from rare to medium in no time. It's all a matter of timing. You know, speaking of timing, that reminds me, Annemarie, my secretary, was telling me today that her daughter just got her period. I know you girls are getting to be that age, and it's something we've never talked about as a family. What've you kids got to say about menstruating. Some wonderful thing, eh?"

"Oh, *Daddy!*"

"Ugh. Right in the middle of the mashed potatoes. Gross."

The zoo, then. One quick trip and you'll be talking sex in no time:

"Mommy, what's that monkey doing?"

"Yes, isn't that sweet, darling. That must be the mommy monkey. She's helping to groom her little baby. She's picking things out of its hair."

"No, not that one. I mean that other monkey."

"Which one? Oh. That one. It's . . . masturbating."

A rule of life says: Whatever can go wrong will. That holds for talking sex as well as everything else in life. Well, thank goodness for good old reliable books.

MEMO TO:	The boys in the back room
FROM:	Your parents
CONCERNING:	Recommended reading
MESSAGE:	It has been brought to our attention by Ms. Martin the librarian that an

error appears on the list of required reading distributed at the end of last Saturday morning's meeting. Ms. Martin reports that *Hot High School Sex Class*, written on the list in orange crayon, does not appear in the library card catalogue or on the list of recommended reading about sex for children at that library. We do not know how this title came to appear on the reading list, and we request that it be removed. Now.

Talking at dinner, watching TV, providing books, taking a trip to the zoo, having a scheduled discussion, even writing letters to your kids—in real life these techniques and limitless others can be used to start a sex conversation. So what if sometimes they backfire, or you end up feeling like a jerk? Life is full of moments—Dr. Lyman Gilmore calls them "teachable moments"—both spontaneous and planned, serious and funny, that can be used to bring up something that a lot of parents find immensely awkward.

"Use opportunities in your child's life," suggests Dr. Zussman. Because talking sex means talking about all the issues involved with sexuality and reproduction and their connection with families and feelings and values, what in life is *not* an opportunity?

Parents who begin to spot the manifold opportunities while their kids are young—the cat's having a litter, the next-door neighbor is pregnant, the baby antelope at the zoo is nursing (or, indeed, the monkey is masturbating)—"then sex becomes just one more natural topic, like radishes growing or buying a new car or anything else," says Dr. Gilmore, "and the kids don't think it's such a big deal."

Television presents more back-to-back teachable moments than probably any other shared family experience in modern life, and sex educators heartily recommend its use as a sex-talk ice-breaker. Certainly you can watch the all-too-few sex-education shows. And you can watch everything else too. The realities and the distortions are both worth talking about.

For young children, television frequently introduces them to situations that are as yet outside their experience. A show about a woman raising a child alone, for example, may introduce the notion that kids don't necessarily have two parents around. Here a parent can take the opportunity to say, in Dr. Zussman's words, " 'This story talks about a different way in which people have families. This baby doesn't have a father living at home. Do you know any children who live in families where there is no father living at home? Of course, a father is needed to start a baby.' " And you can continue into how daddies and mommies make babies.

For the child whose father lives apart from the family, the mother could say, "That's something like our family. Daddy doesn't live here, but did you ever think about how daddy and I got to having a baby together?" Lo and behold, the ice is broken in a real-life way.

TV, and the media in general, are among the best sex-talk facilitators with the older kids, too. They present an especially convenient opportunity to start talking about values and to help kids discern distorted and contradictory messages. For example, everybody on

138 • HOW DO YOU BREAK THE ICE

"Dallas" and the other soap operas has plenty of sex—
but they all seem to have an extraordinary immunity
to herpes and other sexually transmitted diseases. TV
shows and movies that kids watch, ads that they see,
magazines and books that they read, all commonly tend
to equate sexuality and sexiness with physical beauty;
kids who aren't knockouts or who don't think they're
ever going to be could be thinking they're losers in the
sex department. Shows kids like still portray a guy
who's masculine as a guy who "scores." There's no end
to messages the kids are picking up from the media—
not to mention rock music lyrics—that are influencing
their sexuality and attitudes without them necessarily
realizing it. All parents have to do is point these messages out to get an energetic conversation going.

But beware of certain pitfalls. Don't, urges Mary
Lee Tatum, "put down what your child is listening to
or seeing. Instead of saying, 'Why, I've never heard
of anything so ridiculous!' or 'That's just awful!' ask
them what all this means to them and give them pride
in their own critique.

"And if you can do that," she says, "you can go on
to say, 'You know, I'm very concerned about music
and television saying some very irresponsible things
about sex. That just isn't the way life is. In my experience sex has been a wonderful, beautiful part of my
life—but it has always been with consequences.''

TV and rock music represent fantasy worlds, Ms.
Tatum says. The difference between reality and fantasy when it comes to sex is a juicy discussion.

But don't tell the kids to stop listening or watching.
They're going to do it anyway—and your intent is to
break the ice, not to have them freeze you out.

And don't forget the newspaper. Kids have to learn about some of the tougher facts of life too—such as rape and child abuse—and a story in a newspaper is a way to get that going.

For the parent who finds it extremely difficult to talk about sex, even when the opportunity is present, educators and therapists recommend books. There are so many good books about sex aimed at each age group (see the reading list at the end of this book), all you have to do is buy a bunch and leave them around the house along with other books the kids are reading.

These books, of course, are also useful as "supplemental reading" in homes where the subject does come up. "You give the kid the book and then you walk away," says Dr. Gilmore. "Don't bore in with your eyes and insist, 'Now do you have any questions?' because at that point the kid needs to escape. He or she needs to take the book upstairs and giggle over it with friends, or whatever. Kids have to process information about sex in their own way. What you have to do is give them the freedom of their own privacy." Perhaps in a day or two, or next week, they'll come to you with a question.

Say your two cents' worth on the sexual subject you want to bring up, but try not to overdo it. Educators Tatum and Gilmore both mention "the car trick." You've got the kids' attention in the car without other household distractions. And in the car, you can't have eye contact, which helps lighten the embarrassment considerably. Say it and move on to another subject. "It shouldn't be packed emotionally whenever you're giving information. Deliver it off the cuff. And if you can't do it casually," Ms. Tatum recommends, "practice."

Remember that the reason you're trying to break the ice is to create an atmosphere in which the child will feel comfortable about sexual matters and will realize that it's okay to come talk to you "when a question or a problem or a temptation or a crisis comes up," says Dr. Gilmore. Sex should be something that they can talk about in the family—not something they *have* to talk about, or that becomes such a big deal that all other conversation has to grind to a halt.

In other words: try not to put the child on the spot.

Feeling concerned that your ten-year-old son might be suffering some anxiety about masturbating? Don't, says Dr. Lief, go up and ask, "Do you masturbate?" Demanding information invariably "comes across as if the parent will be disapproving. Take the child aside —it should be one on one," he adds, "and say, 'At your age most kids have some concern about masturbating.' This way, too, you universalize the behavior." You relieve the child of the feeling that he's the only kid in the world who does this.

This type of technique takes kids off the hot seat at all levels of sexual development and allows them to see you as trustworthy people who really understand what they're going through. Kids approaching puberty are frequently extremely confused about their changing bodies and feelings. The ice-breaker at this age is to focus on "issues that deal with sexual development," Dr. Cassell says, "the way they look, the way they feel, perspiration, menstruation, nocturnal emission. They really would much rather know more about what's happening to them than about sexual intercourse."

How do you talk about these issues? "You put your

arm around your eleven-year-old son," she says, "and you say, 'Goodness, you are really growing up. I wasn't prepared for this talk for at least five years, but you're getting to be a man. I can see that right now. And you know some of the things that happen when you become a man? During the middle of the night you're going to have an ejaculation. Some people call that a wet dream. This is because . . . ' and you can go into a little biology.

"It's okay to be clumsy," she says. "Kids forgive easily for that." They may giggle and carry on, but they appreciate that you care enough to try.

According to Dr. Schreiner-Engel, commenting on your child's changing body is an excellent way to start a sex conversation even if you've never brought the subject up before: "There is always something changing as a child is growing up, from height to weight to shape. To a daughter, for example, a parent can simply say, 'Gee, I see your body is changing, your hips are growing larger. Have you started getting pubic hair yet?' It's very easy to comment about the body in a very natural way."

The major difficulty for parents of adolescents in trying to start a sex conversation is staying on the right side of the privacy issue. Kids this age usually don't want to talk about anything, let alone sex. Don't push it. "You can express your concerns without insisting that the child tell you something that he or she might feel most reluctant to reveal," Dr. Lief believes.

But by all means, tell them what's on *your* mind. Dr. Cassell thinks a good place to do that is a restaurant. Take your teenage child out to lunch; it makes the child feel important, and it takes you both out of the house and away from your usual relationship. Then look across the table and spit it out. "Why fool around with it?" asks Dr. Cassell. "There's not a single teenager who doesn't know a parent's getting ready for a biggie here. Kids are immediately receptive to straight talk. What they're not receptive to is the double talk: 'Get home on time!' 'What have you been doing?' 'I want you home to do your homework,' and so forth. Kids would rather have you say, 'Look, I'm really afraid you're going to have sex and that you can't handle it.' You're not delivering a moralistic lecture here. You, the parent as a person, are telling them why sex is such a powerful thing."

And if a kid clams up? Ask if he or she would like to talk to anybody else—to the other parent, to an uncle, a teacher, the family doctor—about bodies and emotions and feelings and relationships, because sometimes it just helps to talk these things over with someone. "You want to give the child permission that it's okay if that person isn't you, that you won't feel rejected if he or she would prefer to talk to someone else," Dr. Zussman suggests.

Other ice-breakers? If your relationship with your adolescent is enduring some bad moments, write a note and stick it in a good sex book. Use mealtimes. "The dinner table is a great place for sex talk," Dr. Gilmore declares. "It got to the point in my own family where I could come home and say, 'Did you see this article about sex in *Time* magazine?' or 'One of my students asked me this question today.' And my daughter would roll her eyes up to the ceiling and say, 'Oh, Dad, not *again*.' But you know, you don't have to sit down and have a hard talk about sex."

IN TALKING SEX WITH YOUR KIDS? • 143

It gets easier, the experts say. Once you begin to see how many "teachable moments" there are to start a talk, you may even begin to enjoy yourself. Sex is fun too, you know!

How Do You Break the Ice in Talking Sex with Your Kids?

    A. Schedule a talk
    B. Turn on the TV
    C. Bring it up at dinner
    D. Go to the zoo
    E. Give them books to read
  *F. All of the above

There are plenty of opportunities to talk about sex. Don't be afraid to seize them. All you have to do is sit down with your child and turn on the TV. Sex relates to everything in life—to values and feelings as well as to physiology. If you remember that, talking sex needn't be such a big deal. Once you begin breaking the ice, it get's easier and more natural. Kids don't mind if their parents are embarrassed; it helps them feel okay about their own embarrassment.

Talking sex with your kids is a gift from you to them. It will help them be at ease with sex, starting with that first question: "Hey! Where did I come from?"

Reading List

Recommended books to share with your kids:

Boys and Sex. Wardell Pomeroy. Delacorte Press, 1981.
For early teens.

Facts About Sex for Today's Youth. Revised Edition. Sol
Gordon. Ed-U Press, 1979. For early teens.

Girls and Sex. Wardell Pomeroy. Delacorte Press, 1981.
For early teens.

Growing Up Feeling Good. Ellen Rosenberg. Beaufort
Books, 1983. For preteens.

How Was I Born? Lennart Nilsson. Delacorte Press, 1975.
For young children.

Love and Sex and Growing Up. Eric W. Johnson and
Corrine B. Johnson. Bantam, 1979. For preteens.

Period. JoAnn Gardner-Loulan, Bonnie Lopez, and Marcia
Quackenbush. Volcano Press, 1979. For preteens.

Where Did I Come From? Peter Mayle. Lyle Stuart, 1973.
For young children.